MAKE YOUR OWN
BEAUTY
PRODUCTS

ABOUT CHARMAINE YABSLEY

Charmaine is a freelance journalist specialising in health, nutrition, fitness and beauty. She writes for national newspapers, magazines and websites in the UK and Australia.

She is the author of several health and wellbeing books, including *Naturally Beautiful*, *The Happy Plan*, and the bestselling *Miracle Juices*.

She lives in Australia on the Gold Coast, Queensland with her husband and two sons.

MAKE YOUR OWN
BEAUTY
PRODUCTS

Charmaine Yabsley

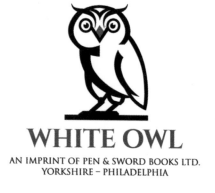

WHITE OWL
AN IMPRINT OF PEN & SWORD BOOKS LTD.
YORKSHIRE – PHILADELPHIA

First published in Great Britain in 2021 by
Pen & Sword WHITE OWL
An imprint of
Pen & Sword Books Ltd
Yorkshire – Philadelphia

ISBN 9781399001625

Printed and bound in India by Replika Press Pvt. Ltd.
Design: Paul Wilkinson

Pen & Sword Books Limited incorporates the imprints of Atlas, Archaeology,
Aviation, Discovery, Family History, Fiction, History, Maritime, Military, Military
Classics, Politics, Select, Transport, True Crime, Air World, Frontline Publishing, Leo
Cooper, Remember When, Seaforth Publishing, The Praetorian Press, Wharncliffe
Local History, Wharncliffe Transport, Wharncliffe True Crime and White Owl.

For a complete list of Pen & Sword titles please contact:
PEN & SWORD BOOKS LIMITED
47 Church Street, Barnsley, South Yorkshire, S70 2AS, England
E-mail: enquiries@pen-and-sword.co.uk
Website: www.pen-and-sword.co.uk

Or
PEN AND SWORD BOOKS
1950 Lawrence Rd, Havertown, PA 19083, USA
E-mail: Uspen-and-sword@casematepublishers.com
Website: www.penandswordbooks.com

CONTENTS

INTRODUCTION

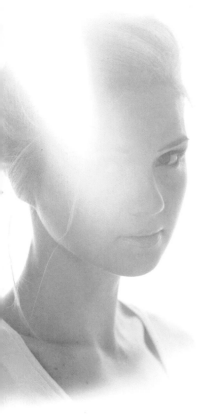

(Courtesy of Gabriel Brandt)

BEAUTY IS BIG BUSINESS. In the UK alone, the beauty industry is worth £1.15bn a year and is expected to grow by 15 per cent in the next five years. Yet the products we use may be causing us harm. And costing us and our environment, the earth.

A large part of this growing market is the consumer demand for clean, natural and organic products: according to the Soil Association Certification Organic Beauty & Wellbeing Market Report, there was a 23 per cent year on year growth of certified organic beauty and wellbeing products sold during 2019. And it's expected to get even bigger.

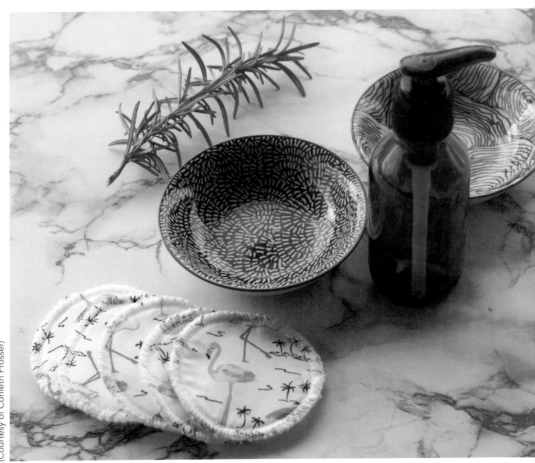

(Courtesy of Conleth Prosser)

This is where *Make Your Own Beauty Products* comes in. This practical and informative guide gives you all the information you need to be as naturally beautiful and environmentally conscious as possible. You'll learn which herbs can be used to soothe, moisturise or repair skin conditions, which vegetables work well as a toner, and how to make rejuvenating masks with your leftover fruit and vegetables.

We'll get you started with a suggested planting guide, to ensure you have a continual supply of ingredients to use in your beauty products. Even if you only have a kitchen garden, aloe vera, mint and chamomile are important elements to include in your beauty regime.

Our easy-to-follow recipes use ingredients which are easily sourced and simple to prepare. And our shopping list will also help you ensure your fridge and cupboards are stocked with all you need.

Whether it is a shampoo, conditioner, facial spritz, cleanser or hydrating mask, our DIY guide will help rejuvenate your skin, while helping you do your part for the environment, and your overall health.

You've shunned packaging, have a small, but flourishing, herb garden, filter your own water and religiously use your recycled shopping bags. But what about your beauty regime? As we begin to embrace a slower, greener and more natural way of life, perhaps it's time to explore the different ways you can include a more natural beauty regime into your life. Which is good news for your skin and overall health. The trend for making your own beauty items is no longer considered 'hippyish' or 'alternative'.

The rise in DIY beauty, and natural beauty, has grown exponentially during the past decade. It's estimated that 41 per cent of beauty consumers use a DIY product (facial cleansers are the most popular). According to Euromonitor International, people are turning towards brands

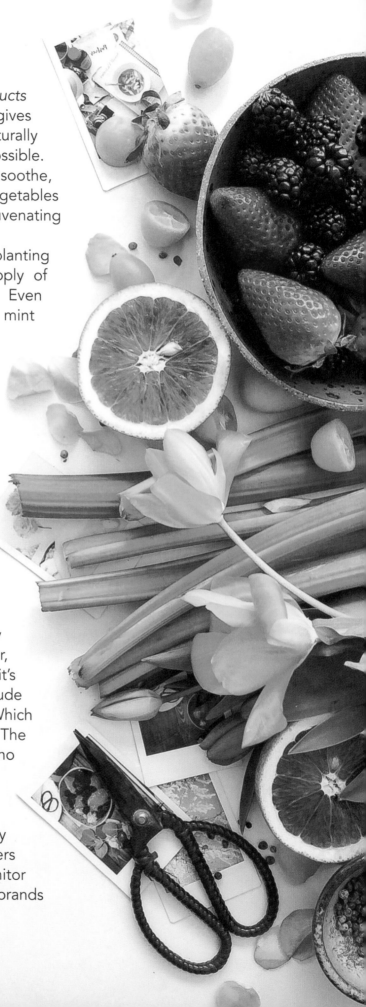

and products that promise transparency. There's also the sense of control you have over what you're putting on your skin, in the same way many of us like to have control over what we consume. It's all about going back to basics.

It's not surprising that there has been a slow but growing backlash against commercial beauty products. In 2019, Johnson & Johnson, the makers of various skincare products – namely baby shampoo and talcum powder – were ordered to pay millions of dollars to a group action, claiming the talc caused their cancer. Another, less publicised court case, agreed with a class action filed by people who blamed haircare company Wen for their hair loss. Fine? $26 million.

Which is where this book comes in. Making your own beauty products means that in the long run you'll save money, plus you'll also know exactly what you're putting on your skin (and in small ways, your body). Which is a positive step for you, your skin, your overall health, and the environment.

CHAPTER ONE

ABOUT YOUR SKIN

THERE'S A GOOD reason why so much research and money are invested in caring for your skin. It is, after all, the body's largest organ. It's a temperature gauge of whether we're happy, sad, hot, cold, feeling hormonal, stressed, tired, whether our system is overwhelmed or dealing with too much sugar, fats or packaged foods.

The skin covers the entire surface of the body – about 18 square feet in all – and is self-repairing and self-renewing. It acts as an interface between your internal and external environment: consider the spots you get around your chin when you're hormonal. That's your internal system communicating through one way it knows how to – your skin.

If you've ever suffered from a skin condition, or breakouts, you know how self-conscious it can make you. By learning about your skin, what it reacts to (both negatively and positively) and what helps to calm it, you're able to take control of your skin's health. After all, like it or not, our appearance is the first thing people notice about us. Eating well, using natural, calming and kind beauty products on our skin are surely the best ways to make a good first impression.

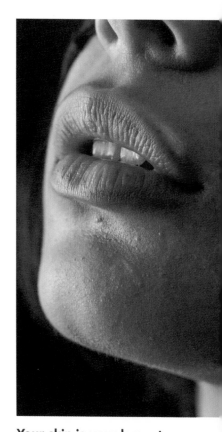

Your skin is your largest organ and can tell you what's really going on with your health, and even your moods.
(Courtesy Engin Akyurt/Unsplash)

HOW OUR SKIN WORKS

It sounds far-fetched to think that a product we apply to our cheeks may have an adverse effect on our organs. But here's how it works:

The skin is made up of several layers. The lowest, the dermis, is composed of connective tissue, blood vessels, nerve endings, hair follicles, and sweat and oil glands. The top layer, the epidermis, is the one that's visible and lies on top of the dermis. Its thickness varies with age, sex, and the body area (for example, the epidermis on the underside of the forearm is about five cell-layers thick, but on the sole of the foot it might be as much as 30 cell-layers deep).

Under the dermis is the subcutis – or the hypodermis. This is composed of a layer of fat (known as adipose) and fibrous tissue.

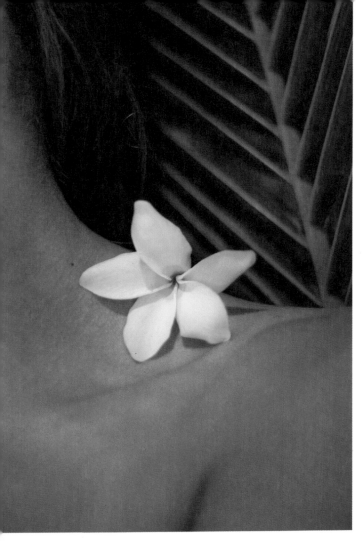

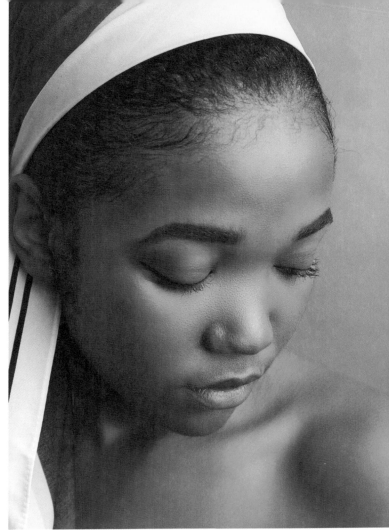

Our skin is made up of several layers. It's important to eat well and use natural ingredients for healthy looking skin. Courtesy Andrey M Hackson/Unsplash)

Following a beauty regime – cleanse, exfoliate, tone and moisturise – is the best way to achieve gorgeous, glowing skin. (Audrey M Jackson/Unsplash)

Every person's subcutis is different, depending on their size and weight. This layer is responsible for protecting the body from trauma, insulating your body from the cold and storing energy.

Our skin tells us a lot about our environment. Cold, or scared? You'll get goosebumps. If you're hot it helps to stop you from overheating; too cold and your inner body temperature will help warm you up and your skin will constrict and small hairs will raise up to trap any emanating warmth. Conversely, when we're overheated, our skin becomes relaxed and sweat comes out of our pores. For the most part, our skin is impermeable to water, but will absorb some moisture (this is why our skin wrinkles when we're in the bath, pool or ocean for too long).

As we age, our skin becomes slower at renewing itself, which is why it's so important to regularly cleanse and exfoliate our skin. By removing the dead skin cells, the skin underneath can breathe and properly absorb the goodness of our beauty products. When our skin is in good health, it's able to protect our body (and health) from external elements, such as free radicals – including environmental toxins, and pollutants, harmful bacteria, viruses, parasites, pathogens, antigens and UV radiation.

The epidermis renews itself every 15–30 days. Interestingly, if you have psoriasis (characterised by red, itchy rashes), the skin is renewed every 7–10 days.

Our skin is also the dustbin for our bodies. Sounds lovely, doesn't it? But as our largest organ, our skin is the conduit for the removal of toxins. Clear, clean pores expel chemicals and waste easily. If your pores are clogged, or you have a build-up of products on your skin, then your skin can't do its job properly. The result? Breakouts, skin irritations and rashes.

One of the reasons natural beauty products are so important and helpful for your skin is that they help it maintain its healthy layer of protective oils. Using soaps, moisturisers or body scrubs which contain harsh chemicals can remove and deplete our body's natural protective oils, leaving it open to infection or skin problems.

WHAT OUR SKIN DOES – A LIST

- Protects against water loss
- Defends the body against physical and chemical injury. And bugs!
- Helps our body fight allergens, toxins and carcinogens
- Heals wounds
- Regulates our body's temperature
- Protects us from the UV rays of the sun
- Allows us a sense of touch, feeling and pleasure
- Skin produces vitamin D which helps prevent many diseases including osteoporosis, cancer, hearts disease, obesity and neurological diseases

UNDERSTANDING YOUR SKIN TYPE

Not all skin is created equal. Knowing the type of skin you have, and in particular knowing what can trigger a reaction is an important step in your self-care and beauty regime.

If you're confused about what type of skin you have, here's an easy way to find out. First thing in the morning wipe a piece of white paper over your skin (be careful of paper cuts!). If the piece of paper has:

- No oil marks = normal or combination skin
- Oil marks = oily skin
- Nothing, but you could feel your skin drag = dry skin
- Made your skin feel sore = sensitive skin

Knowing your skin type can help you eat the proper diet to support it and use the correct products so that you're not doing more harm than good.

WHAT IS YOUR SKIN TRYING TO TELL YOU?

It is possible to look at your reflection and determine several health issues, whether it's dehydration, overburdened liver or kidney, or hormonal issues. Always check any sudden or unusual skin changes with your doctor.

Skin issue	Cause
Sudden breakouts	Stress and anxiety.
Puffy eyes	Lack of sleep, too much time in front of devices or computer, or a salt-heavy diet.
Pimples, acne or breakouts along jawline	Hormonal issues such as polycystic ovarian syndrome (PCOS).
White patches	Anaemia (it could also be an indication of other illnesses so it's best to check this out with your GP).
Dark circles under eyes	Nutrient deficiency and dehydration.
'Butterfly'-shaped rash	Lupus or rosacea (again, check with your GP).
Yellowish eyes	High cholesterol.
Dry skin	Underactive thyroid.
Yellow bumps on arms and legs	Early indicator of diabetes.
Pimples around nose and mouth	Digestive issues or food allergies/sensitivities.
Pimples around chin area	Sensitivity to dairy or hormonal issues.
Sudden appearance of wrinkles	Too much sugar in diet.
Flaky skin (including scalp)	Zinc or vitamin B deficiency.
Brown patches on face	Melasma – caused by a change in hormones (tends to appear during pregnancy but fades after the birth).
Cracked lip corners	Iron deficiency.

CHAPTER TWO

INGREDIENTS TO AVOID

THERE IS AN ugly side to your commercial and store bought beauty products: their contents. It's estimated that your stash of beauty products contains more than 5,000 chemicals – and many of these are thought to cause harm or skin and health issues.

A report by the non-profit Environmental Working Group (EWG) found that most women use 12 products containing 168 unique ingredients every day. Men, in comparison, use 6 products daily with 85 unique ingredients. And while the jury is still out on the long-term effects of all these ingredients, it is believed that 1 out of every 13 women and 1 out of every 23 men are exposed to ingredients that are 'known or probable, human carcinogens every day through their use of personal care products'.

Some of the most problematic ingredients in your beauty products may appear innocent in the contents list. Words such as propylene glycol, mineral oil, alcohol, petrolatum, isopropyl myristate, triethanolamine and glycerine do not benefit the skin in any way and may even have long-term harmful effects.

Your skin, the body's largest organ, absorbs up to 60 per cent of the ingredients in your body products. It makes sense then to keep your self-care products as natural and 'clean' as possible. When your skin absorbs an ingredient, it eventually lands in your bloodstream. Many chemicals accumulate in specific organs, or are metabolised through your system, before being dispelled or dissolved – a process which may take several years.

Some health issues which are associated with specific ingredients that are commonly found in many self-care items include endometriosis, endocrine issues, early puberty, thyroid issues, and obesity, amongst others.

Even so-called commercial 'natural' products which claim to be organic or use wholesome ingredients may not be all they seem to be. For instance, the words 'lemon extract' in your shampoo does

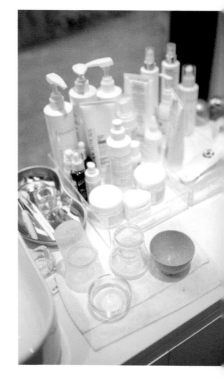

Many commercial beauty products contain ingredients which may not suit your skin, and are harmful to your health and the environment.
(Courtesy Polina Tankilevitch/Pexels)

not necessarily mean pure lemon juice has been added during production, but a synthetic replica may have been used instead. The best way to check if a store-bought product is truly natural is to check the label. Ingredients are listed in descending order, with the largest quantities included listed first.

PARABENS

Your body absorbs up to 60 per cent of the ingredients in your beauty products.

(Courtesy Hana Brannigan/Pexels)

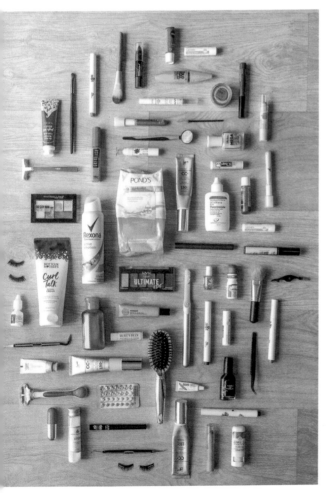

You've probably heard of these bad guys – they're a preservative found in beauty and skincare items such as creams, lotions, deodorants and body wash. Beauty companies put them into products to help prolong their shelf life, preventing the growth of bacteria and mould. While research is still ongoing, it's believed that parabens can penetrate the skin's surface, nestling within the tissue. This can cause problems, as it's believed parabens disrupt hormone function by mimicking oestrogen. When you have too much oestrogen in your body, health issues can occur – parabens have been linked to breast cancer and reproductive issues. Some studies indicate that parabens may also lead to premature ageing and DNA damage.

What to look for: butylparaben, methylparaben and propylparaben are the most common names for parabens.

PHTHALATES

You may have read a lot about the dangers of phthalates, as they've received a lot of negative press over the past decade. Phthalates are found in hundreds of household items, children's toys, pill coatings, flooring, packaging, medical devices, fragrances, lotions and shampoos.

But what are they? Put simply, the chemicals act as binding agents and also make plastics flexible. There has been extensive research into the side effects of phthalates on our health, which is where the advice gets a little blurred. Health issues such as asthma, attention-deficit hyperactivity

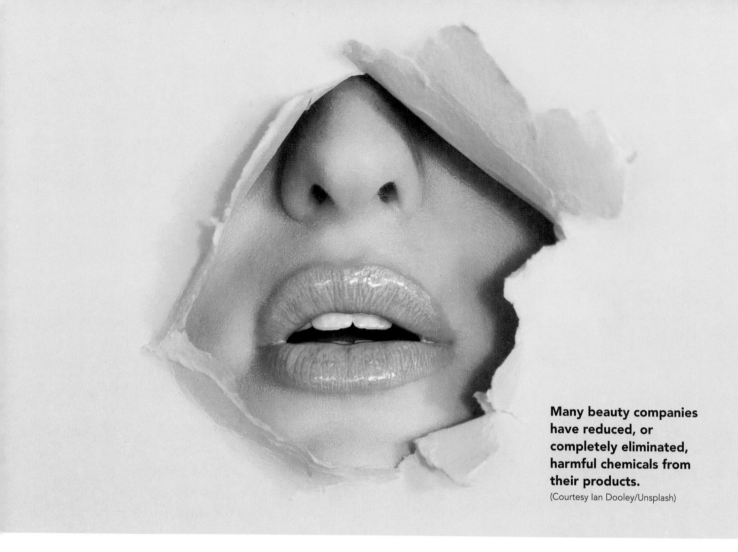

Many beauty companies have reduced, or completely eliminated, harmful chemicals from their products.
(Courtesy Ian Dooley/Unsplash)

disorder, breast cancer, obesity and type II diabetes, low IQ, neurodevelopment and male fertility issues have all been linked to the presence of these chemicals in our daily products.

The good news is that during the past few years many companies have made a concentrated effort to eliminate or reduce toxic chemicals, including phthalates, from their products.

What to look for: Dibutylphthalate (DBP), dimethylphthalate (DMP) and diethylphthalate (DEP) are the main culprits, although since 2010 DEP is the only one still commonly used in cosmetics.

> ∽ **FACT** ∽
>
> Research shows that women have higher levels of **phthalates** in their urine then men.

ETHYLENE OXIDE

This preservative – a solvent – is used in many cosmetic and personal care products to help preserve them, preventing spoiling. However, the jury is still out on the long-term negative effects of it, namely its role in breast cancer cases.

Ethylene oxide is in a wide range of cosmetics and hygiene

products, including perfume, foundation, blush, lipstick, soaps, hand sanitiser and ultrasound gel.

Concerns over its safety are wide reaching, particularly in 2008 when the US Food and Drug Administration (FDA) recalled a product called Mommy Bliss – a nipple cream which contained the solvent – over concerns of its effects on the central nervous system of breastfeeding infants. Studies also show that the presence of this ingredient can cause allergic and skin reactions.

LEAD

You may have heard the rumour that women eat between 3 and 10lbs of lipstick per year. Although this isn't strictly true, the reason many women are worried about ingesting their makeup is because lipstick contains, alongside many other ingredients, traces of lead.

While the amount of lead in lipsticks is almost miniscule and is considered too small by the FDA to be of a health concern, it's the accumulation of lead in the body which rings an alarm.

In one report, 'A Poison Kiss', it was found that exposure to metals in cosmetics, such as the lead in lipstick, have been linked to health issues including reproductive, immune and nervous system toxicity.

What to look for:

Lipsticks which contain mica (a naturally occurring mineral that adds shine to lip gloss) contain metals such as lead, manganese, chromium and aluminium. Typically, the deeper, or stronger the colour, the bigger the metallic load.

TRICLOSAN

If you brush your teeth, then you've most likely used a product containing triclosan. Added to many consumer products to reduce or prevent bacterial contamination, triclosan is mostly found in antibacterial soaps, body washes,

> **✎ FACT ✎**
>
> On average, women reapply their lipstick up to twenty-nine times a day.

If you chew your lipstick off, don't worry, you're not going to do your body any long-term harm.
(Courtesy Shiny Diamond/Pexels)

toothpastes and some cosmetics. It can also be found in clothing, kitchenware, furniture and toys.

Further human studies need to be done in order to find out the full- and long-term effects of triclosan. Tests on animals have raised concern over this ingredient due to the findings of decreased thyroid hormones and increased resistance to antibiotics.

What to look for:

If you're concerned about your product containing triclosan it will be marked clearly on the 'ingredients' list on the label.

SKIN DEEP – INGREDIENTS TO BE WARY OF

Chemical	Commonly found in	Known side effects
Phthalates	Deodorant, perfume, nail polish, synthetic fragrances	Linked to breast cancer, early puberty in girls, diabetes and obesity in children, diabetes
Parabens	Creams, lotions, deodorant, body wash	It's believed that 75–90 per cent of cosmetics contain parabens These have been linked to breast tumours.
Ethylene oxide	Shampoo, perfume, moisturisers, creams	Linked to an increase risk of breast cancer
Lead	Lipstick, nail polish, toothpaste, foundation, sunscreen	Reduces fertility. Has been linked to language delay and learning and behavioural problems.
Triclosan	Deodorant, toothpaste, soaps, body wash	Hormonal disrupter, may affect thyroid and metabolism

CHAPTER THREE

SKIN ISSUES

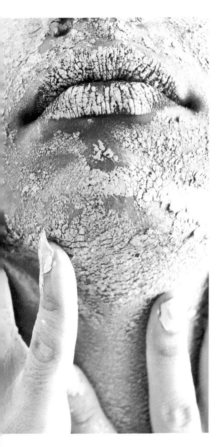

Knowing what works for your skin will help eliminate any nasty reactions or breakouts.
(Courtesy of Ricardo Garcia/Pexels)

HOW TO TREAT SKIN PROBLEMS, WHAT TO EAT, WHAT TO AVOID

No matter how old you get, you'll probably face some skin problems. Whether it's teenage breakouts, dry skin, pregnancy patches or wrinkles, caring for our skin is a lifelong task! Knowing how to treat certain skin issues, through topical treatments and diets, can go a long way in reducing the emotional and physical effects that skin issues can cause.

ACNE, BLEMISHES, BREAKOUTS

Acne – or acne vulgaris to give it its proper name – doesn't just affect teenagers. Anybody can get acne: the red, sometimes painful bumps which can appear anywhere on your face, although largely around the chin, cheeks and forehead. (The back, neck and chest can also be afflicted.)

So what causes it? There are two main causes: when the sebaceous, oil-producing glands block the hair follicles and pores, bacteria build up and spots or acne can form. In teenagers, this tends to occur because the hormones, which control the sebaceous glands, are working overtime. Some women may find that they suffer from acne during pregnancy, or when they're menstruating – again due to hormonal fluctuations.

HOW TO TREAT IT

One of the best remedies for acne, and indeed any skin condition, is zinc. It's a powerhouse of a mineral; enhancing immune function, reducing inflammation and promoting healthy hormone levels. Zinc helps skin growth, so it's essential for those suffering from acne, as it helps to heal outbreaks and may also prevent further blemishes. Another supplement or food source to consider is vitamin B6, which helps to regulate hormone levels (ideal if your acne is worse at times of menstruation, puberty, pregnancy or menopause). Foods rich in essential fatty acids (EFAs) should be eaten at every meal, as they help reduce the amount of oily sebum that can clog pores.

What to eat:
While it's easy to assume that anybody with acne has a poor diet, this isn't necessarily true. What is known is that a good, balanced diet, full of fruit, vegetables and lean meat and fish is ideal. It's believed that a low-fat, high-fibre diet can help prevent breakouts, but also reduce healing time. Foods rich in vitamin A, such as eggs, liver, fish and oils, are thought to help the skin heal. Vitamin A is also found in skin treatments, such as Retinol, a well-established treatment for acne.

Drink filtered water – at least 1.5 litres a day. Adding collagen drops or lemon juice can add taste, but also help encourage better skin condition and appearance.

What not to eat:
Research shows that diets high in sugar may exacerbate acne, and some people find that dairy products can also make their blemishes worse. If you do suffer from acne, try cutting dairy from your diet for a week or two to ascertain if it's a culprit.

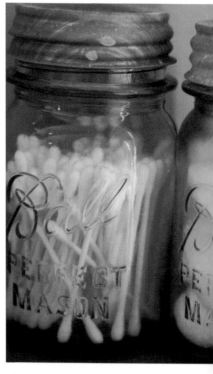

If you have a pimple or blemish treat it with natural solutions and keep it hydrated.
(Courtesy of Jen Theodore/Unsplash)

AGEING

It happens to everyone at some point, but there are ways to help reduce the appearance of lines, age spots and damaged skin which can make you appear older than you really are. While there's nothing wrong with ageing in years, taking care of your skin to help it appear as healthy as possible is recommended. Glowing, smooth skin tends to be associated with youth, but there's no reason people of all ages can't boast a radiant complexion.

Ageing, or changes to your skin appearance – less smooth or even in tone – is caused by loss of elastin and collagen in the skin. As we get older, our skin becomes thinner, so when we repeatedly make facial expressions (whether it's smiling or frowning) these create creases that over time become permanent.

One of the biggest contributors to ageing is the sun. Every time

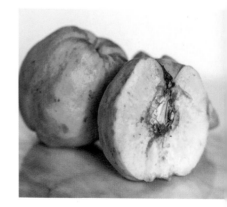

There's nothing you can do about the passing of time, but you can help your skin look as clear and healthy as possible – whatever your age.
(Courtesy of Alex Loup/Unsplash)

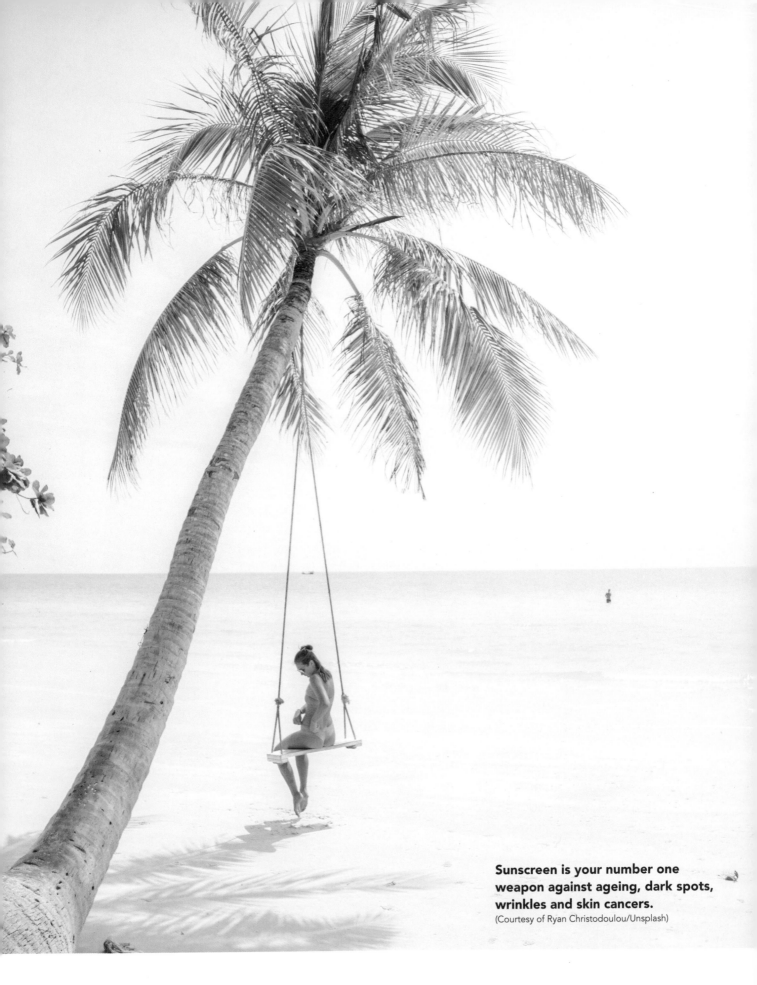

Sunscreen is your number one weapon against ageing, dark spots, wrinkles and skin cancers.
(Courtesy of Ryan Christodoulou/Unsplash)

you get sunburnt, or 'tanned' you're doing damage to the skin. The two main ultraviolet rays – UVA and UVB – damage the skin in several ways. Repeated exposure to UVB rays causes short-term damage to the epidermis and long-term damage to the deeper layers and skin tissue. UVA rays penetrate the skin more deeply than UVB rays and alter the structure of the elastic fibres in the dermis. They also exacerbate damage caused by UVB rays and speed up the photo-ageing process.

It's imperative to wear sunscreen every day, regardless of the weather. The higher the sun protection factor (SPF) the better the protection. Experts recommend wearing an SPF of at least 30, applied thirty minutes before going into the sun.

Many face products – moisturisers and foundations – now contain SPF, although it's not recommended you rely on these items alone to protect your skin. According to the Skin Cancer Foundation, most cosmetic formulations lack enough protection against UVA rays, which are present year-round and can even travel through window glass.

Instead, always apply a broad spectrum lotion (this means it protects you against UVA and UVB rays) every morning, after your serum and moisturiser. Remember though, no matter how high your SPF, no sunscreen will protect your skin for more than two hours. Reapplying sunscreen won't afford you another two hours, so it's best to seek shade instead. Don't forget the tip of your nose, ears and neck, which are often forgotten and prone to sun damage.

A good rule of thumb: your SPF number applies to the 'times greater' protection it gives you. For instance, SPF30 gives you 30 times better protection than without, SPF 50 gives you 50 times the protection. And check the ingredient list. If it contains zinc oxide it will reflect UVA and UVB rays from the skin's surface – it's also an ideal treatment for pimples and acne.

Don't forget: environmental factors, such as smoking, sun rays and pollution are the biggest causes of premature ageing. There are no products which can permanently turn back the hands of time, taking good care of your skin every single day goes a long way to helping it appear at its best.

What to eat:
Foods which contain antioxidants help strengthen your skin's layers against pollutants and external factors which can cause ageing. Hero

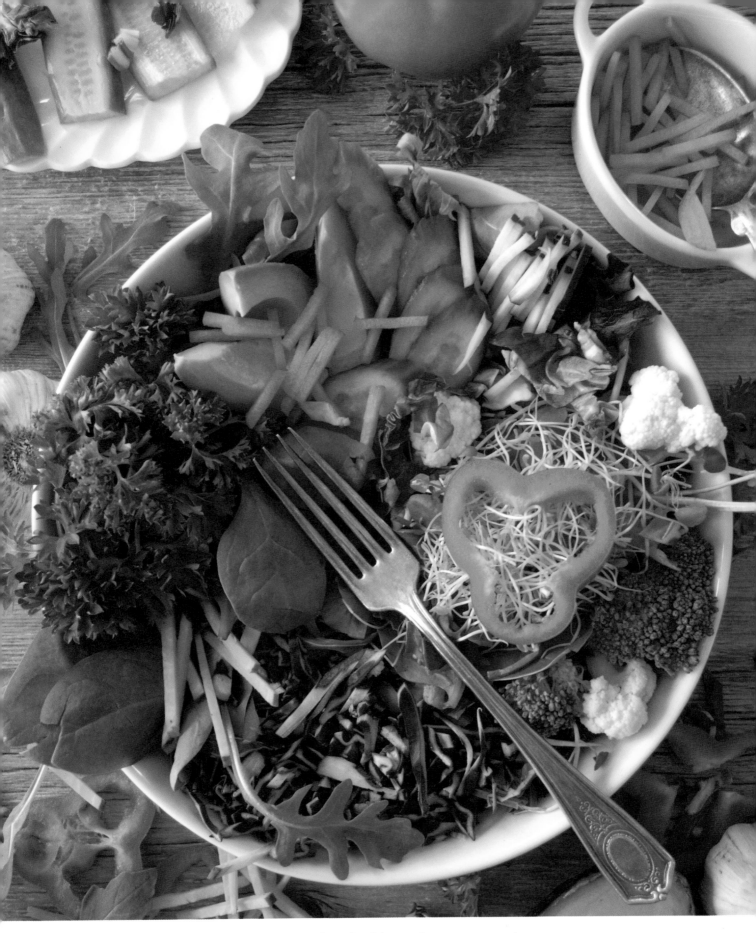

What you eat is just as important for your skin's health as what you put on it. (Courtesy of Nadine Primeau/Unsplash)

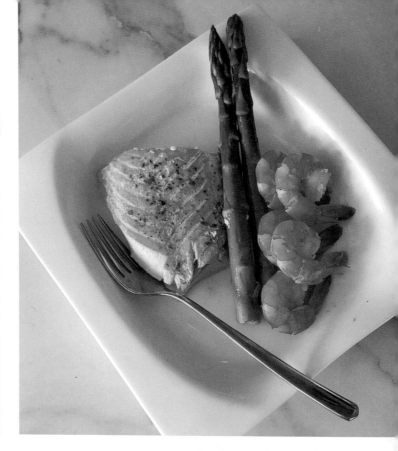

TOP TIP

Cut the sugar! Not only is sugar bad for your waistline and gives you false energy, but a more-than-healthy sugar intake can cause ageing and uneven skin tone. When you eat sugar it attaches to protein in your bloodstream and produces harmful free radicals called advanced glycation end products (AGEs). The more AGEs you accumulate, the more damage they can cause to the proteins around them. These proteins are important as they provide the foundation for collagen and elastic – the stuff that makes your skin plump and firm. It can also encourage the appearance of brown discolouration marks and age spots.

Feed your skin foods rich in omega-3 essential fatty acids.

antioxidant foods include carrots, squash, spinach and broccoli. Aim to eat your recommended 5–7 daily servings of vegetables every day to get your full antioxidant load.

Dry, dehydrated skin wrinkles more easily, and can make your skin look older than it is. Other than drinking at least 2 litres of water a day, foods rich in omega-3 essential fatty acids can help 'plump' up your skin. Salmon or shellfish are great EFA-rich foods. Alongside omega-6, which is found in nuts, seeds, sunflower oil and wheatgerm, these EFAs help to reduce inflammation, which can affect the rate your skin's cells are renewed. Unchecked, this can lead to premature ageing.

DERMATITIS AND ECZEMA

Around 1–3 percent of people suffer from eczema and research shows that it's on the rise. According to Allergy UK, eczema is a common skin condition in babies and infants but can also occur in older children and adults.

Eczema is when there is a breakdown of the skin barrier, which can lead to exposure of allergens via the skin, resulting in the production of IgE antibodies and the development of an allergy.

Some people find that hormones, stress or certain products can exacerbate the problem, leading to patching of red, hardened and usually, painful skin areas.

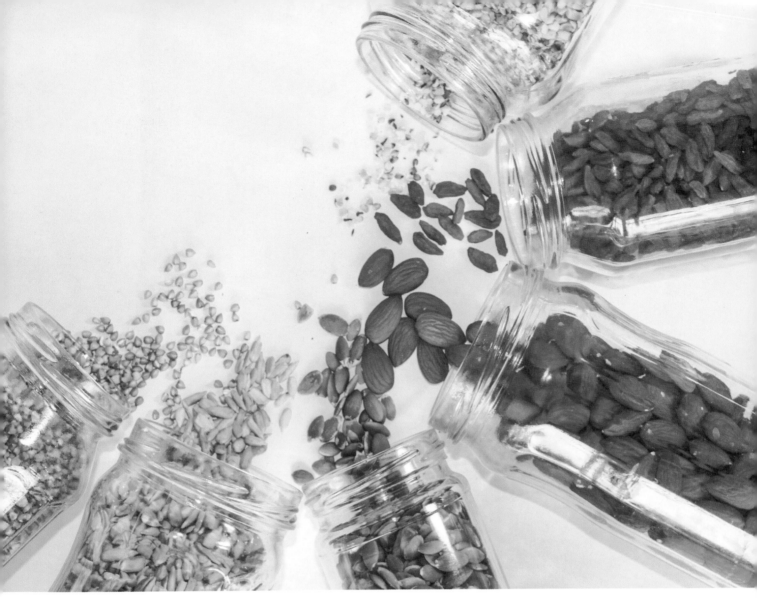

Dry, itchy or allergy prone skin needs extra attention. A diet rich in healthy oils is a must.

What to eat:

Foods containing beta carotene and vitamins C and E have been shown to help calm inflamed skin, reduce inflammation and itchiness.

If your skin has flared up, and it's feeling dry and itchy, counteract these with carrots, avocado, spinach, sweet potato, sunflower seeds, pine nuts, herring and anchovies. A strong and healthy immune system may also help reduce your skin's tendency to breakout – so load up your plate with zinc foods such as pumpkin seeds, beef, lamb and sardines.

What to avoid:

For some people kiwi fruit is a godsend for their irritated skin, packed full of vitamin C. However, others react badly to it. Unfortunately, unless you have a specific skin allergy test, it can be a case of hit-and-miss when it comes to trigger foods. Generally, common culprits include milk, eggs, shellfish, wheat, chocolate, nuts and strawberries.

DRY SKIN

If your skin feels taut, tight or appears dull, it could be that you have dry skin. The good news is that you're probably less likely to have breakouts. On the other hand, dry skin can become flaky, look older than it is, and may be prone to redness or itchiness.

Dry skin occurs when the sebaceous glands don't release enough sebum to keep the skin lubricated. Sebum, alongside natural oils or lipids and natural moisturising factors, forms a barrier called the hydro-lipid system. This barrier helps your skin maintain its moisture levels – however, if you don't have enough of these natural moisturising factors, then your skin can appear dry.

What to eat:

Water really is your friend when it comes to dry skin. Foods with a high water content are also ideal – think cucumber, watermelon, peppers. Foods that contain vitamin B may also help reduce water loss in your skin, along with vitamin E which helps to neutralise free radicals that can cause skin sensitivity and dryness. Find vitamins B and E in wheatgerm, cod, turkey, beef, bananas and mango.

TOP TIP

If you have dry skin, then it's extremely important to avoid extreme temperatures, such as heating or hot water. Never put your face directly in the hot water stream in your shower (use a flannel or face wipe instead).

If there's one change you make to your beauty routine make it the amount of water, and foods which contain a high water content, you drink.

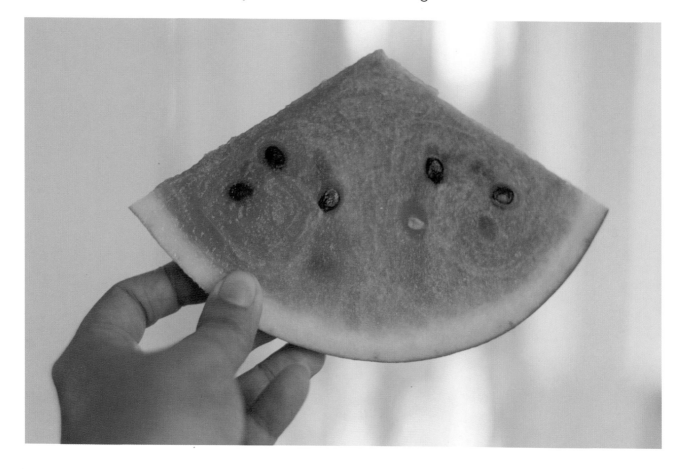

CHAPTER FOUR

AN A–Z GUIDE OF BEAUTY FOOD

YOU KNOW THE saying, 'You are what you eat'? Never a truer word was spoken when it comes to your skin's health.

It's not rocket science. Eating a well-balanced diet, with a focus on organic fruit and vegetables, fish and lean meats, plenty of filtered water and limited sugar and caffeine are good building blocks for optimum skin health. There are certain foods which provide more benefits to your skin than others, and some ingredients which will undo all your good work!

And what makes a fruit or vegetable beneficial for your diet, and ultimately your skin, can also have topical powers too. Read on to find out which foods you should include in your daily meal plans, and some tips on how and why we use them in our DIY beauty recipes too.

Your skin will quickly show the effects of a bad – and good – diet. Feed your face with healthy, organic food as much as possible.
(Courtesy Brooke Lark/Unsplash)

APPLE

An apple a day certainly keeps the skin doctor away. They're a great source of vitamins C and E, which are antioxidants that help produce free radicals. (Free radicals are the nasties caused by a poor diet, smoking, pollution and stress.) Antioxidants are a vitally important part of your diet as they help the skin's cells renew and repair themselves. You know when your skin is looking grey, tired and lifeless? That's a sign that your diet needs a good input of antioxidants.

If you're getting spots around the mouth, this is an indication that your bowels are a little sluggish. Boost your fibre intake, which apples have in abundance. Apples also contain malic acid, which is believed to help reduce the appearance and formation of cellulite.

❧ TOP TIP ❧

Eat your apples with the peel on, as this is where the majority of the nutrients lie. However, you can use an apple peel as a soft exfoliant. Simply rub the inside of an apple peel over your face, wash with cool water and apply moisturiser as usual.

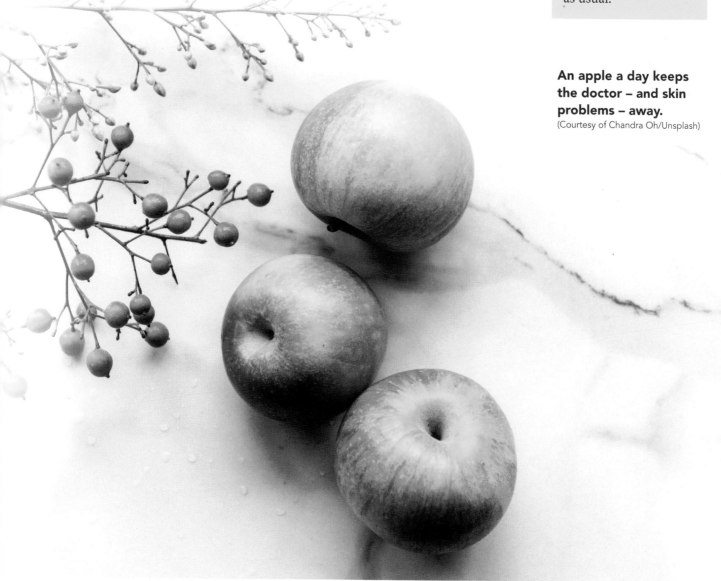

An apple a day keeps the doctor – and skin problems – away.
(Courtesy of Chandra Oh/Unsplash)

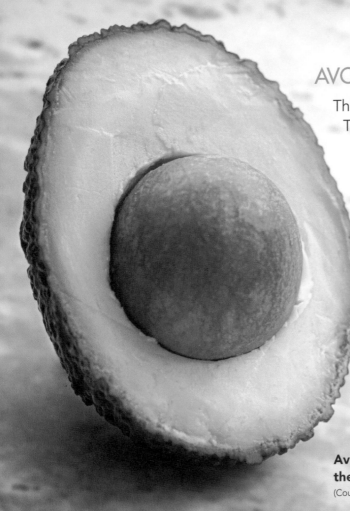

AVOCADO

These fruits are truly the stars of the beauty world. They're ideal for topical use and are also one of the best ingredients to include in your diet. They're packed with healthy fats (which help your skin look smooth and plump) and vitamins A and E. The monosaturated oils in avocados help to maintain the integrity of the membrane which surrounds your skin cells. One study found that women who boasted supple skin also had a diet with a high intake of healthy fats found in avocado.

If you're prone to inflamed skin conditions, such as eczema, acne and psoriasis, then including avocados in your diet may help. The presence of vitamins A and E help the skin to produce new cells too, the secret to a glowing appearance.

Avocados are a must for your natural beauty cabinet. Eat them, use them as a face mask, or a hair treatment.
(Courtesy of Mali Maeder/Pexels)

BANANA

Bananas are full of potassium, which helps promotes cellular growth and also keeps any puffiness at bay, so they're ideal to eat after a long flight or a workout when you're likely to be dehydrated.

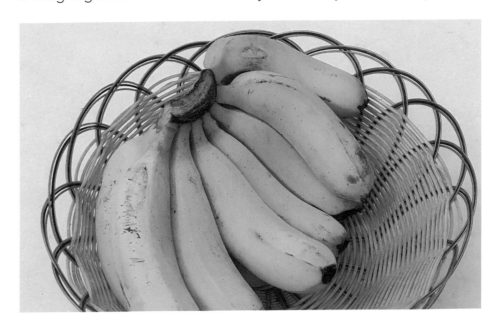

Bananas are ideal to give you energy, but can also treat many skin issues.
(Courtesy of Syed Hussaini)

They're also rich in vitamins A, B and C, all of which are necessary for helping to boost moisture, promote cellular growth and prevent ageing.

And they're not just for banana bread. Using banana in your beauty recipes means that you'll be adding some great moisture into your skin or hair.

BEETROOT

These wonderful root vegetables are often forgotten about – possibly because they're fiddly to cook (especially without staining yourself and your worktop). However, persevere with them, as they're packed full of skin- and health-boosting goodness. They contain large amounts of nutrients and vitamins, including iron, vitamin C, folate, fibre and potassium. Beets also contain anthocyanins, members of the flavonoid family, which have anti-inflammatory and antioxidant properties. Beetroot, and beetroot juice, when eaten or drunk, have been found to help those with acne, and may help prevent signs of ageing.

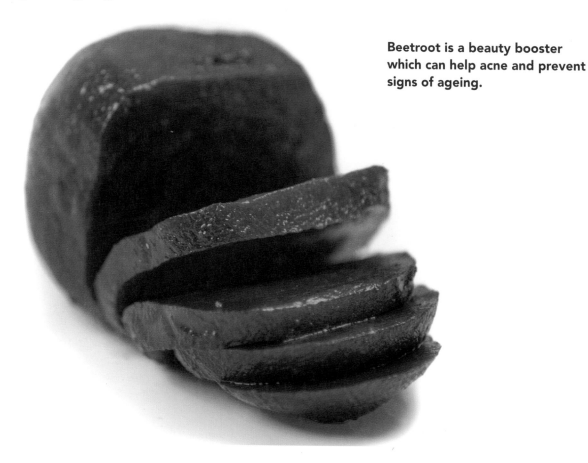

Beetroot is a beauty booster which can help acne and prevent signs of ageing.

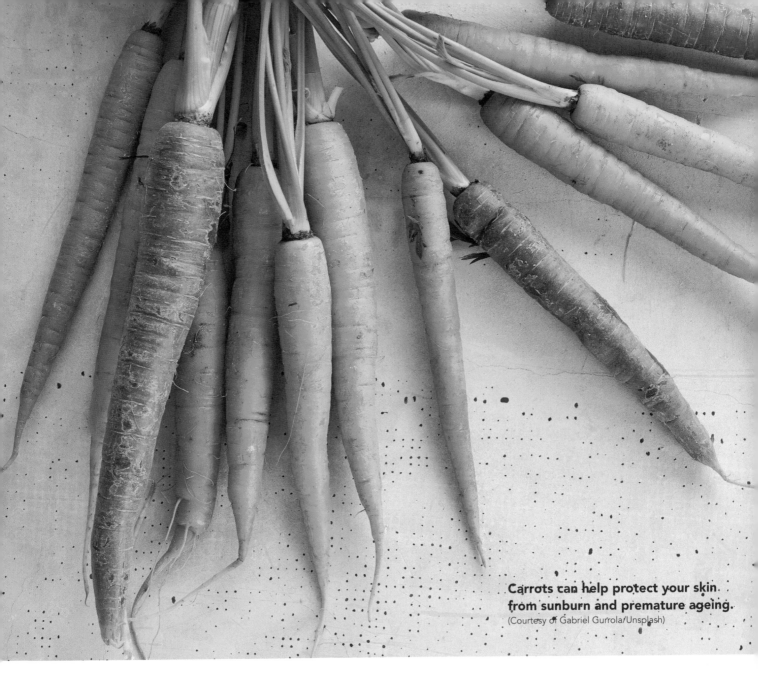

Carrots can help protect your skin from sunburn and premature ageing.
(Courtesy of Gabriel Gurrola/Unsplash)

❧ TOP TIP ❧

Sweet potatoes are an excellent source of beta carotene too. Replace your usual potato-based meals with sweet potato instead. They're much lower in carbohydrates and fat and a great source of vitamin E, ideal for those suffering from eczema or psoriasis.

CARROT

Bugs Bunny's favourite snack should be yours too. Packed full of healthy beta carotene, it works as a natural skin booster and sunblock, helping to protect your skin from sunburn, premature cell death and dry skin. (You still need to wear sunscreen daily, but carrots are a good way to help boost your skin protection from the inside.)

Many skin products contain carrot juice, or an extract of carrots, due to their high vitamin C content and natural antiseptic properties.

DID YOU KNOW?

Ancient Greek folklore believed eating carrots helped increase sexual appetite.

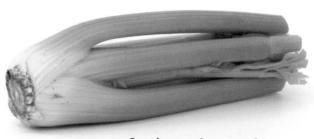

CELERY

Great for snacks, and adding extra crunch to a salad, celery isn't just for those watching their waistline. With a water content of up to 95 per cent, it's great for hydrating your skin, it's also recommended if you've overdone it with the sugar and alcohol, as it may h e l p support the kidneys as they rid these toxins from your body. Healthy kidneys mean strong, supple skin, so try to add some celery to your daily salad. Recently, people have championed the health benefits of plain celery juice – it's not particularly tasty, so I'd stick to adding it to salads and your beauty recipes.

Snack on celery as often as possible. It's great if you're watching the calories, plus it'll add to your day's water intake.

∾ TOP TIP ∾

If you do juice your celery keep the pulp as it's a great face mask (see page XX).

COCONUT OIL

This wonder oil is definitely a must for your cupboard. Whether it's cooking with it, or using it as a base for your recipes, or even just as a moisturiser on its own, coconut oil is an integral part of natural beauty – inside and out.

Made from extracting the oil from coconuts and dried coconut kernels, it's rich in saturated fat and medium-chain fatty acids. What

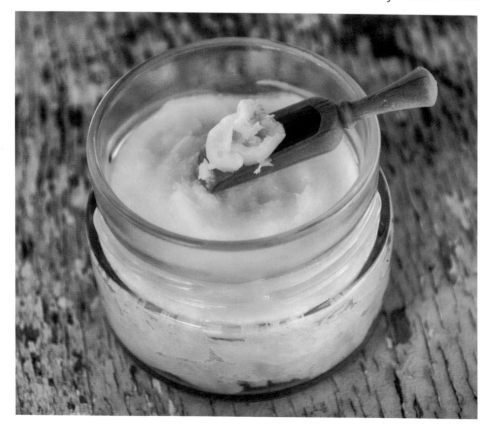

You can cook with it, eat it, bathe in it, and use it for many beauty treatments. Coconut oil should be in your kitchen and your bathroom cupboards.

(Courtesy of Biome.com.au)

If you suffer from athlete's foot, skin infections, or acne, applying coconut oil directly to the affected area may help banish bacteria and speed up the healing process.

does this mean for your health? Despite its popularity, experts warn against overloading the coconut oil when cooking. It's high in saturated fat, which can lead to heart disease, so use it sparingly, or better yet save it for your beauty regime.

Using coconut oil as a moisturiser has many health benefits, in particular if your skin is inflamed, or you have psoriasis, contact dermatitis or eczema. The anti-inflammatory properties of this oil have been found to help improve the appearance of these skin conditions and soothe it too.

CUCUMBER

If you've ever placed cucumber slices onto tired or puffy eyes, then you're probably already aware of the cooling and anti-inflammatory benefits of these vegetables.

Internally, cucumbers are helpful for your skin, due to their high water content, helping to improve your hydration. Adding slices of cucumber to your filtered water may improve the taste if you don't like to drink it plain.

Using cucumber juice has long been part of a natural beauty routine. Alongside its use as an eye treatment, you can also use the juice for a cleanser, toner or to reduce redness caused by irritation or sunburn.

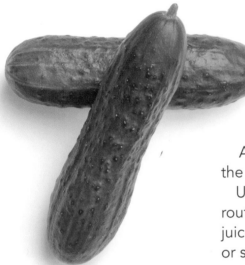

Cucumber is a wonderfully cooling toner for red or inflamed skin. (Courtesy of Unsplash)

HONEY

This great cupboard staple is also ideal for inside and out skin treatments. Taken internally, honey can help relieve a sore throat (due to its anti-bacterial and anti-inflammatory properties). It also contains iron, which is necessary for optimum skin cell growth and healthy looking skin. A spoonful of honey a day may also support your digestion – when this doesn't work properly your skin can reflect this with congested pores, particularly around the chin and nose.

Honey is a great healer – for sore throats, spots or dry lips.
(Courtesy of Danika Perkinson/Unsplash)

Dry, flaking lips? Apply some honey to your lips and leave it for at least twenty minutes. Then, take a toothbrush and softly remove the honey. This will exfoliate flaking skin without ripping the delicate area.

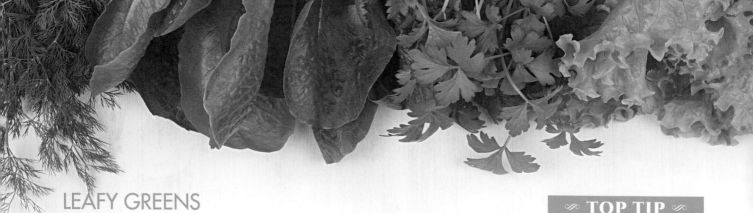

LEAFY GREENS

Leafy veg, such as lettuce, kale, spinach and watercress are all wonderful additions to a healthy eating plan. They have a high water content, plus they contain iron, vitamin C and beta carotene. These are necessary for cell-renewing and ensuring well-nourished skin. Eating these leafy greens can help your nails become stronger, as they're a good source of folate which promotes nail and hair growth.

LEMON

Almost every diet tip includes adding a squeeze of lemon to your water. Why? Some experts say that it helps internal cleansing and kick-starts the digestive system, which in turn keeps blemishes at bay (a clogged digestive system can lead to mouth and chin spots). These sour fruits are high in vitamin C, which plays a vital role in the formation of collagen – the 'scaffolding of the skin'. As we age, our collagen levels drop, which leads to wrinkles and duller looking skin. Topically applied vitamin C may help reduce signs of ageing, sunspots and wrinkles.

TOP TIP

Using lettuce in your DIY beauty routine may seem a little strange but it's actually a wonderful toner and cleanser as it can help to restore your skin's pH levels and reduce redness.

Lemon is a natural astringent – use it to banish cold sores, dry out spots and improve your digestion.

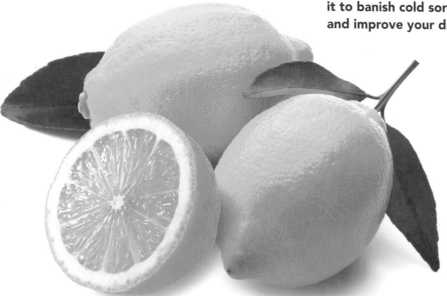

TOP TIP

Squeeze some lemon juice over your spinach salad to help your body increase the absorption of iron and vitamin C.

Nothing says summer like a ripe mango. Add it to your morning cereal or fruit smoothie for a delicious start to the day. (Courtesy of Pixabay/Pexels)

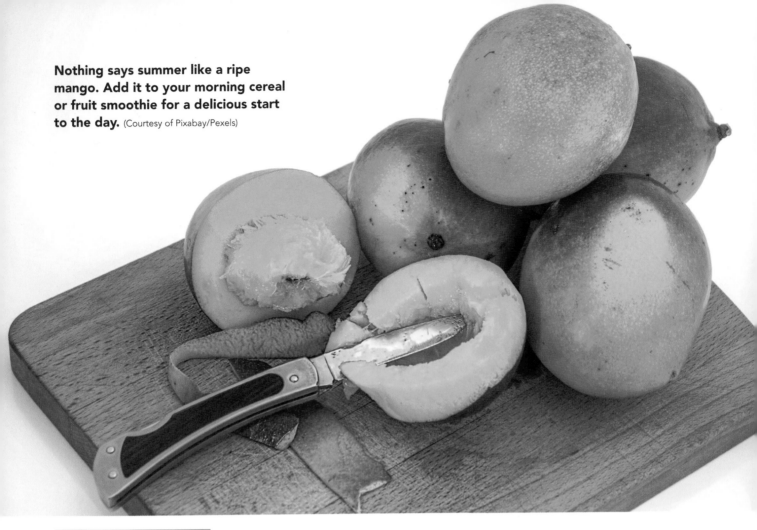

∽ **TOP TIP** ∽

A mango smoothie with some added yoghurt is ideal to help support kidney function, leading to a smooth, glowing appearing skin.

MANGO

I always associate mangoes with hot summer days when the juice runs down your chin and there's joy to be found in the mess! These stone fruits are rich in antioxidants, vitamins B3, C and E, and beta carotene. When you eat beta carotene, it is converted into vitamin A in the body – this is essential for healthy skin.

MELON

∽ **TOP TIP** ∽

Applied to sunburnt skin, melons really come into their own, helping to soothe heat rash, acne or blisters caused by too much sun.

Whether it's watermelon, rockmelon, honeydew or cantaloupe, the health and skin benefits are the same. Rich in phytochemical lycopene and beta carotene which help protect your skin against skin cancer, these fruits are ideal for summer eating. They also all have a high water content, so enjoy them as part of your hydration regime.

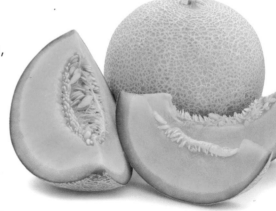

Melons are ideal summer foods to enjoy for plump, smooth and hydrated skin.

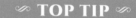

Olive oil has numerous benefits and uses. You can use it in your recipes, both to eat and to apply to your skin.

OLIVE OIL

The Mediterranean diet is widely regarded as the healthiest diet in the world, citing lower cases of heart disease, cancers, obesity and high cholesterol as its benefits. One of the heroes of the diet is, of course, olive oil.

Olive oil is recommended for a healthy gall bladder and liver, regular bowel movements and a healthy digestion. When these organs are working optimally, your skin tends to be clear and healthy. However, a build-up of toxins can lead to dermatitis, eczema, psoriasis, rosacea, acne and general breakouts. Vitamin E is present in olive oil – internally, this helps promote skin elasticity and healing. One word of warning: don't use too much olive oil when cooking or on salads, as it's still high in fat. Keep to around two tablespoons a day.

PINEAPPLE

If your skin takes a little while to heal, you may need to add some pineapple into your diet. Pineapple contains bromelain which helps to treat peeling or blemished skin, and aids in speeding up the healing process. It's ideal to eat after a big meal too, as it supports the digestive system by helping to break down proteins in the stomach.

Pineapple contains alpha-hydroxy acids (AHAs), a term or acronym you've probably seen on your exfoliant or anti-ageing creams. AHAs are widely used within the beauty industry, as they help to gently remove dead skin, making way for new skin cells to appear and grow. They're also included in anti-ageing products as research shows that regularly use of AHAs can help reduce the appearance of fine lines, wrinkles and sun and age spots.

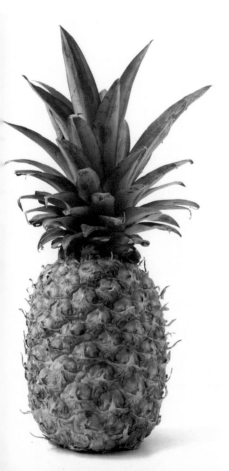

Pineapple can help speed up the healing process – it's ideal for acne prone skin.
(Courtesy of Miguel Andrade/Unsplash)

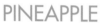

❧ **TOP TIP** ❧

Olive oil is a good base for massage oil or moisturising your face, body and hair.

❧ **TOP TIP** ❧

If you don't have skin allergies, then you can apply a piece of pineapple directly to your skin to slough off any dead skin cells.

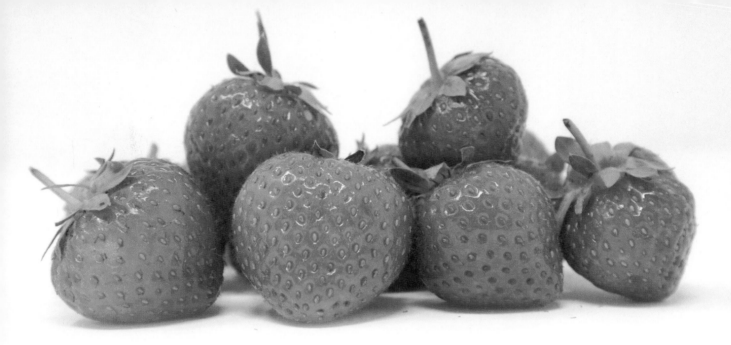

Rub strawberries against caffeine stained teeth to reveal your lovely white pearlers. (Courtesy of Frederick Tubiermont/Unsplash)

STRAWBERRY

These wonderful berries – an icon of true love – contain the antioxidant vitamins A, E and K, so they're ideal if you have a skin condition or inflammation. And they're perfect for ageing skin, as the vitamin C is crucial to the formation of collagen. If you suffer from fine lines, or have notice tiny red capillaries appearing on your skin, then add some strawberries to your morning muesli or smoothie. Once again, the star vitamin C can help reduce the appearance of these capillaries and prevent more forming.

If you suffer from acne, consider increasing your daily intake of strawberries (around a handful is ideal). These small red fruits help to cleanse your digestion, ridding the body of any toxins which may lead to skin eruptions.

TOMATO

Packed full of beta carotene, tomatoes are also an important part of the Mediterranean diet due to their high antioxidant levels. They provide around 40 per cent of an adult's recommended daily intake of vitamin C, so they're a must when it comes to keeping skin supple and smooth. When eaten, tomatoes can help protect the skin against free radicals, reducing premature ageing and skin damage, particularly from the sun and

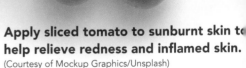

Apply sliced tomato to sunburnt skin to help relieve redness and inflamed skin. (Courtesy of Mockup Graphics/Unsplash)

TOP TIP

Applying tomato juice to the skin may help reduce irritations or redness caused by sunburn.

external elements. Some research shows that eating tomatoes may offer some protection against sunburn – however, it's better to wear a high SPF and include tomatoes into your daily diet.

OATS

If you keep one staple ingredient in your cupboard, make it this. You can eat oats or use them as a face mask, eczema treatment or body scrub. Dietary wise, oats are great for energy, as they're a complex carbohydrate. They're also full of protein – twice as much as brown rice. And if you suffer from seasonal affective disorder (SAD) then try to have oats – such as porridge – as often as possible for breakfast. They'll help to boost your serotonin levels and ward off depression and low mood.

❧ **TOP TIP** ❧

Oats can help relieve feelings of stress which may lead to an outbreak of spots, particularly along the jawline.

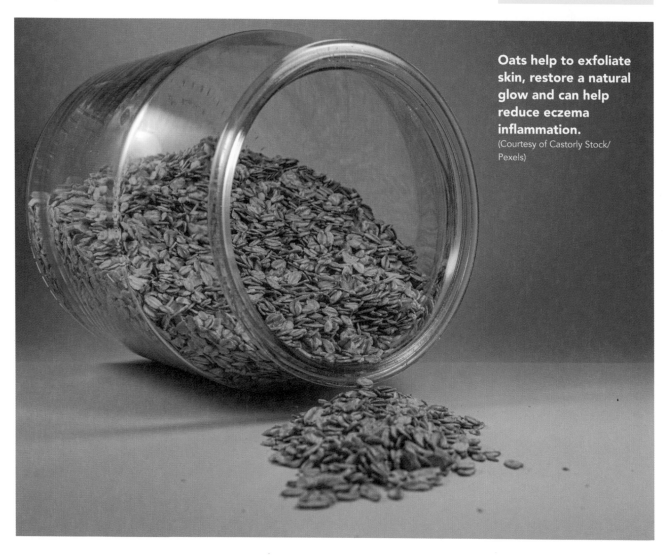

Oats help to exfoliate skin, restore a natural glow and can help reduce eczema inflammation.
(Courtesy of Castorly Stock/Pexels)

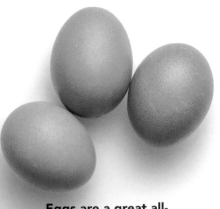

Eggs are a great all-rounder. Use them for face masks and include them in a healthy, balanced diet.
(Courtesy of Melissa DiRocco/Unsplash)

EGG

Remember the ad campaign 'Go to work on an egg'? There's a good reason it was embraced. Eggs help build strong bones, and through their vitamin D, help boost immunity and ward off low mood. If you've been worried about cholesterol levels, research has now concluded that eating one egg a day brings a large array of health benefits, with no risk of heart disease. Eggs also contain zinc, lysine, vitamins A and E, and biotin, all of which are needed for the growth and repair of healthy skin cells, to prevent white spots on nails and promote hair growth.

YOGHURT

Along with the oats in your cupboard, always keep yoghurt in your fridge for both health and beauty benefits. Eating yoghurt may be one of the secrets to optimum health, as it contains the friendly bacteria needed that may help prevent diarrhoea, constipation and irritable bowel syndrome (IBS).

Yoghurt is a great inner and outer beauty ingredient to use for optimum gut health and reduce red, irritated skin conditions.
(Courtesy of Burst/Pexels)

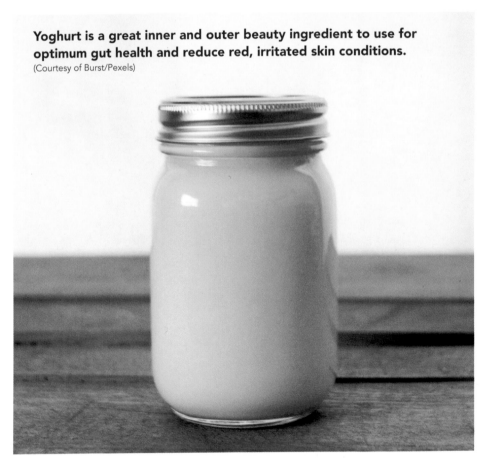

YOUR HEALTHY SKIN DIET – AT A GLANCE

SKIN TYPE	WHAT TO EAT
OILY	**Omega-3 essential fatty acids:** linseeds, wheatgerm, trout, soya. **Zinc:** lamb, beef, oysters.
SENSITIVE	**Omega-3 essential fatty acids:** extra virgin olive oil, sunflower and pumpkin seeds, brazil nuts, almonds, spinach, fish, salmon.
DRY	**Vitamin B-rich foods:** milk, cheese, yoghurt. Wheatgerm, cod, turkey, beef, bananas, cabbage, mango, butter, herring, anchovies, avocado.
NORMAL/COMBINATION	**Omega-3 essential fatty acids:** salmon, fish, linseed oil, tuna, sunflower seeds. Also sweet potatoes, carrots, chicken, rice, pork, mango, watermelon.
ALLERGY PRONE – DERMATITIS AND ECZEMA	Carrot, avocado, spinach, sweet potato, sunflower seeds, pine nuts, herring, anchovy, pumpkin seeds, beef, lamb, sardines, green peppers, cabbage, cauliflower, broccoli.
AGEING	Carrots, squash, spinach, broccoli, oily fish – salmon, shellfish – nuts, seeds, wheatgerm.
ROSACEA	Yoghurt, sauerkraut, kefir, miso, bananas, onions, leeks, asparagus, garlic, whole grains.

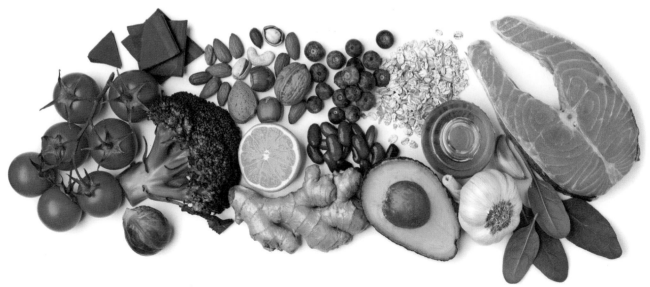

YOUR TOP SEVEN MUST-HAVE BEAUTY FOODS

Not all foods can be applied to your skin, but I still recommend that you consider including these on your regular shopping list, and as part of your inner beauty regime.

1. FATTY FISH

Think salmon, herring, mackerel. If you're a fish lover, then it's likely that you have plump, youthful-looking and glowing skin. Fatty fish is high in skin-boosting omega-3 fatty acids, which are a must when it comes to keeping your skin in tip-top shape. If your skin is dry and flaky (particularly in winter), make sure that you're eating fish at least three times a week to keep your levels high. It's also high in vitamin E, necessary for protecting your skin against inflammation and free radicals.

Fish is ideal for optimum skin, and overall, health.
(Courtesy of Gregor Moser/Unsplash)

> ∽ **TOP TIP** ∽
>
> If you are also taking vitamin E supplements, you can pierce the capsules and use the oily contents to spread over your skin for an immediate deep moisturising treatment.

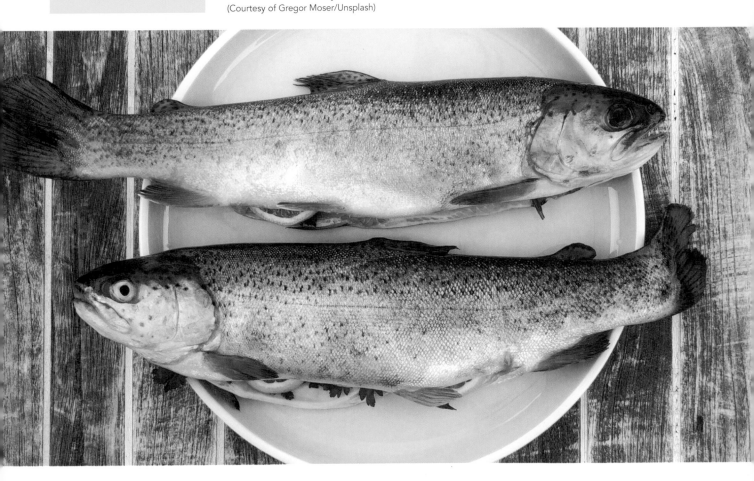

2. WALNUTS

While you'd avoid using walnuts on your skin (they're too harsh, so avoid any products which contain these as they can cause irritation) eating them is one of the best daily habits you can form for your skin, and overall health. They're an excellent source of essential fatty acids – the fats your body can't make – and have the highest amount of both omega-3 and omega-6 fatty acids, compared to other nut sources. Research shows that a diet high in omega-6 fats may help reduce inflammation of the skin, particularly in skin conditions such as psoriasis.

Walnuts are also high in zinc, which is an essential mineral to help your skin function well and act properly as a barrier.

See also: hazelnuts, brazil, macadamia, almonds, pecans, cashew nuts.

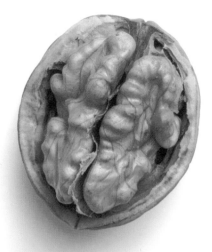

Add walnuts to your salads for a wonderfully healthy boost of oils.
(Courtesy of Mockup Graphics/Unsplash)

> ✎ **TOP TIP** ✎
>
> If you've ever experienced cracks in the corner of your mouth, this can be an indication that your body is low in zinc.

3. SEEDS

While your diet should contain a wide range of nuts and seeds, particular attention should be given to sunflower seeds. Like walnuts, they contain a high level of zinc, so they're great for skin healing. They're also a good source of nutrients, including vitamin E.

Pumpkin seeds are also ideal for salads or adding to breadcrumbs. Also eat: sesame seeds, hemp seeds, linseeds.

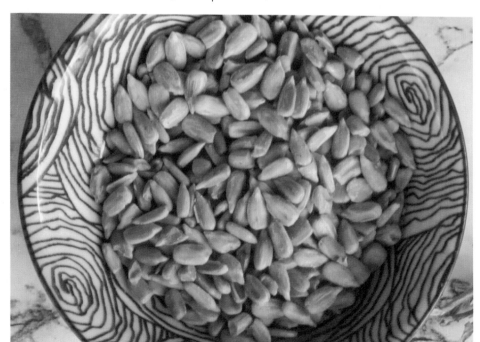

Sunflowers seeds, and other seeds such as pumpkin, sesame, hemp and linseeds are ideal to add to salads, smoothies and fish dishes.
(Courtesy of Conleth Prosser)

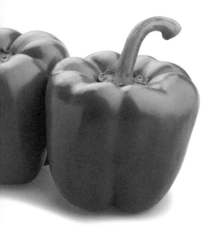

A medium-sized pepper provides more than three times the recommended adult daily intake of vitamin C.

4. PEPPERS (CAPSICUM)

The strong red and yellow colour of these vegetables is down to their high levels of beta carotene, which can be converted by the body into vitamin A. A medium-sized pepper also provides more than three times the recommended adult daily intake of vitamin C – so they're ideal during winter when you're prone to colds and illnesses. They also help boost your collagen levels.

Also eat: pumpkin

5. BROCCOLI

It may be disliked by many children, but this brassica vegetable packs a powerful skin and health-boosting punch. It boasts zinc, vitamins A and C, all of which are a must for optimum skin health. It also has lutein (similar to beta carotene) – used to protect your skin against oxidative damage (the stuff that causes your skin to become dry and lined). The florets of broccoli contain sulforaphane, which is thought to help protect against some types of skin cancers. Again, it's a beneficial food to include in your healthy skin diet.

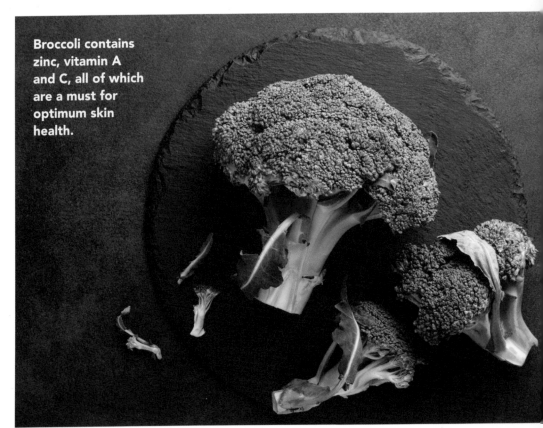

Broccoli contains zinc, vitamin A and C, all of which are a must for optimum skin health.

> ❧ **TOP TIP** ❧
>
> One study found that middle-aged women who ate large amounts of vitamin C had fewer visible wrinkles and dry skin than those who didn't include vitamin C-rich foods in their diet.

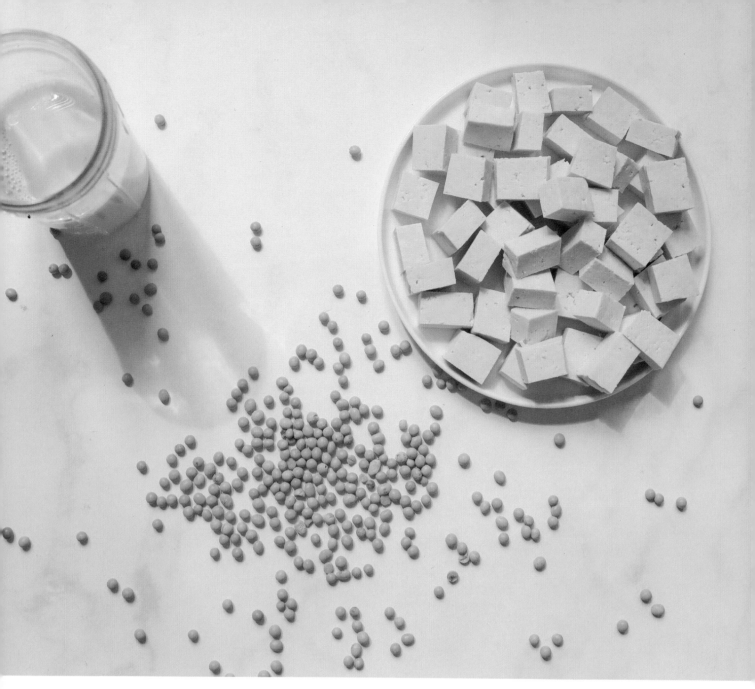

6. SOY

As women age, our bodies produce less oestrogen, which has some knock-on effects on our skin, which loses its elasticity and may appear and feel drier than usual. Incorporating soy or soya beans into your diet is a good way to incorporate isoflavones which help your skin retain its moisture level. One study found that post-menopausal women who ate soy every day for eight to twelve weeks reduced the appearance of fine wrinkles and improved the elasticity of their skin.

Also eat: pulses such as chickpeas, kidney beans, lentils, rice, wheat, rye, beans and peas.

Including soy or soya beans into your diet is a good way to help your skin retain its moisture level.

(Courtesy of Polina Tankilevitch/Pexels)

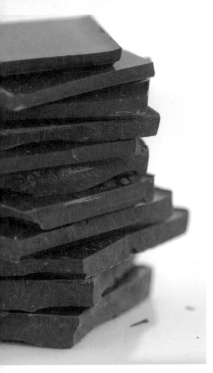

7. DARK CHOCOLATE

The best part of any diet! While highly processed chocolates or sweets are loaded with sugar, numerous studies show that dark chocolate is beneficial for your skin AND your health. Studies show that eating dark chocolate, as part of a Mediterranean diet, has many health benefits due to its high levels of antioxidants.

Chocolate lovers rejoice! Chocolate, particularly dark chocolate, is good for your skin, and overall health. Just keep it to one or two pieces a day.
(Courtesy of David Greenwood Haigh/ Unsplash)

∽ TOP TIP ∽

Eating dark chocolate may help your skin against the harsh rays of the sun. It's believed that the flavanols found in the cocoa beans can help improve blood flow to the skin and increase the skin's density and moisture levels.

WHAT TO DRINK?

Drinking water – up to 3 litres every day – really is the best habit you can make for your skin. Even if you're applying expensive moisturisers and face masks, they'll do little for your skin if you're not hydrated from the inside out.

Your body is 75 per cent water and water is necessary for all bodily functions, flushing toxins through your liver and kidneys and helping to pump oxygen through your body. We tend to drink less water during winter, but if you've got the central heating on you may be inadvertently dehydrating your skin. The good news is that hot drinks, such as tea, coffee, herbal teas, all add to your daily water quota.

As the largest organ in the body, your skin contains around 9 litres of water. When the epidermis – the layer of skin closest to the surface – is well hydrated, the cells are plump and smooth. If you have been neglecting your water intake, your skin will start to become dry and more prone to wrinkles (think of a grape as it dries in the sun).

∽ TOP TIPS ∽

If your face is looking a little puffy it may be that your kidneys need a helping hand. Kidneys filter and neutralise bodily waste: they need water to help them flush toxins and excess out of the body. If you've been eating too much salt this can upset the delicate balance, as your kidneys will reabsorb too much water, leading to fluid retention and puffy-looking skin.

If you're bored of water consider drinking green tea instead. It contains compounds called catechins which help to improve your skin by protecting it against sun damage, helping smooth the appearance of rough or dry skin, and boost hydration levels, which means your skin will look less lined or dry.

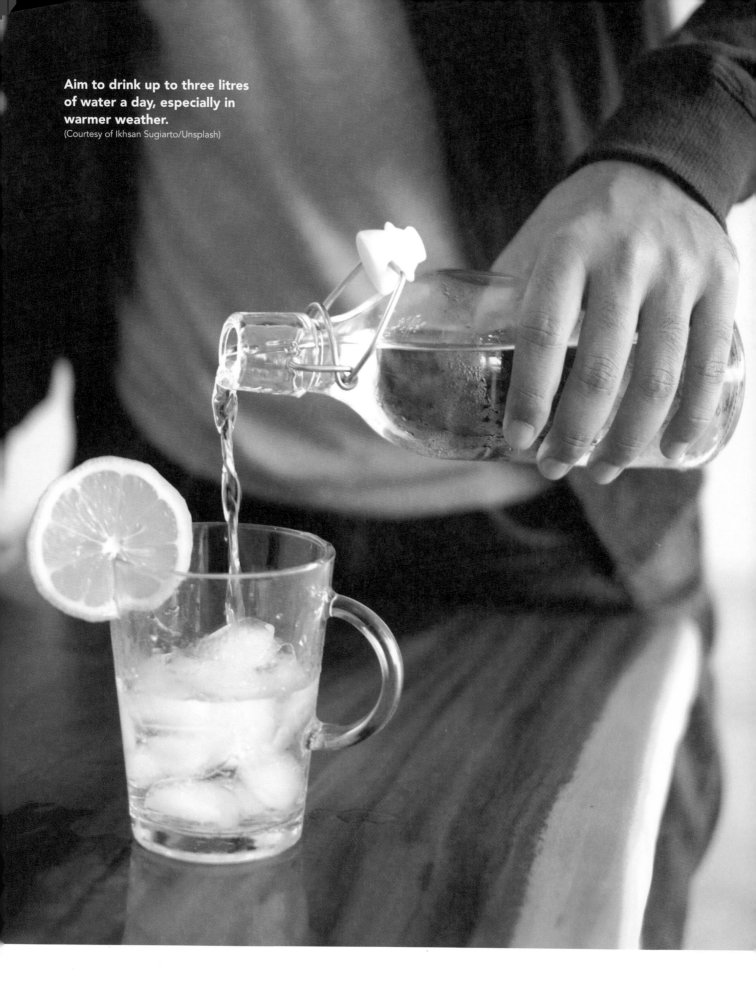

Aim to drink up to three litres of water a day, especially in warmer weather.
(Courtesy of Ikhsan Sugiarto/Unsplash)

CHAPTER FIVE

WHAT TO PLANT FOR A BEAUTIFUL GARDEN

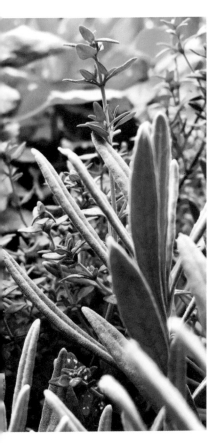

Planting your own herb garden is a great way to include some tasty ingredients in your cooking, and some healing into your beauty products.
(Courtesy of Lisa/Unsplash)

WHAT TO PLANT IN YOUR HERB GARDEN FOR USE IN YOUR DIY FACIAL RECIPES AND MEALS.

One of the benefits of making your own beauty products is being able to utilise whatever is in your fridge or cupboard. You can take this self-sufficiency one step further by planting certain plants and herbs to include. Not only are many herbs a great addition to beauty treatment but you can also add them to meats, seafood or salads, or make healing and calming teas from them. Here's how to get started on your beautiful garden plot.

A good gardening tip is to seek advice from a gardener or expert at the garden centre when buying seeds or plants. Ask for the medicinal variety as these contain the constituents necessary for healing.

Even a small plot of garden, balcony or kitchen can be your herb garden. As long as the area has enough sunlight and you water the plants regularly, you should be able to grow some wonderfully healing herbs to use in your skincare.

ENGLISH LAVENDER (LAVANDULA ANGUSTIFOLIA)

Most people associate lavender with scented pillows and night time. And they'd be right. English lavender is known for its relaxation properties, helping to reduce stress and insomnia.

Another, less well-known variety, is spike lavender (Lavandula latifolia), often used for its antiseptic properties. You can incorporate it into coconut oil and use it on fungal infections, particularly on your feet. (Do not use on children under the age of two years.)

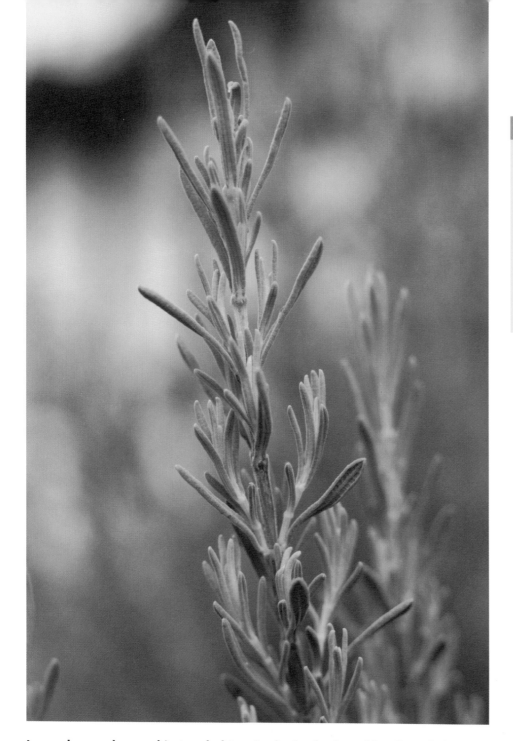

Lavender can be used in tea, baking, in the bathtub and in oils to help promote calm. (Courtesy of Conleth Prosser)

TOP TIP

Tie a bunch of lavender together with some eucalyptus leaves to make your shower smell like a spa (the steam from the hot water will help diffuse lavender's relaxing smell).

If you're making your own soap, grow some Lavandin (Lavandula x intermedia), which has a strong fragrance and is ideal for cleansing.

How to grow: Plant your lavender according to instructions, in a warm, protected spot. You can plant in clumps if you want a burst of colour. Water regularly and trim any woody parts to encourage growth.

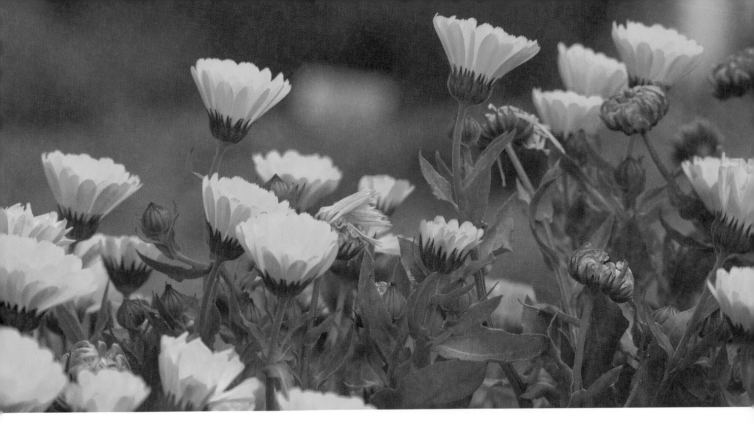

CALENDULA (CALENDULA OFFICINALIS)

Most healing creams contain calendula, which is a wonderfully soothing ingredient that helps heal minor cuts and scrapes. It has anti-inflammatory and healing properties, so it's a good herb to plant for your very own first-aid garden.

Calendula is particularly gentle, so it's ideal to use on children and is often included in even commercially produced nappy rash products.

How to grow: You can grow this herb in a pot or garden. It does attract bees, so it is better if you plant near cruciferous (cauliflower, broccoli, cabbage etc.) vegetables. If you're planting from seed do so after winter, or just before the end of the cold season. Plant indoors, keeping the pot inside for eight weeks.

These flowers are quite hardy so won't need to be watered more than once a week (depending on how dry the climate is where you live). Deadhead flowers to promote growth and cut back if they're beginning to die off. This will give your plants another lease of life.

How to use: When your calendula flowers are fully opened, cut them from the stem and spread them onto a screen or flat tray to dry out. When the petals have turned papery, they're ready to use. You can use them immediately in teas and creams or store them in an airtight jar to be used later.

ஒ TOP TIP ஒ

Sprinkle cakes with calendula flowers for a pretty topping.

ROSE (ROSA SPP.)

Roses not only look and smell beautiful; they have long been used in beauty products for their calming properties and uplifting scent.

How to grow: Plant in pot or along the fence line. You may need to treat roses for disease or insects, although they're quite hardy.

How to use: You can sprinkle some rose petals into a warm bath for a deliciously relaxing scented treat, or add to boiling water, along with lavender, to make a soothing facial spritz.

Sprinkle some rose petals in your bathtub for a gorgeous scented treat.
(Courtesy of Max Berger/Unsplash)

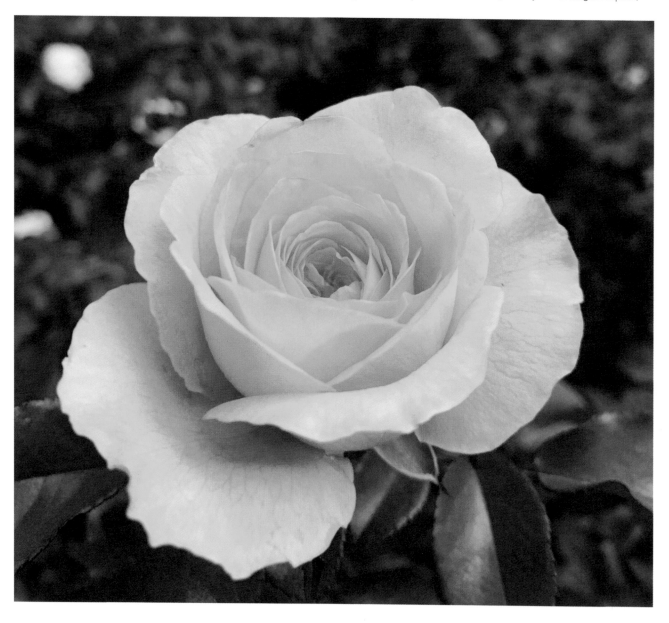

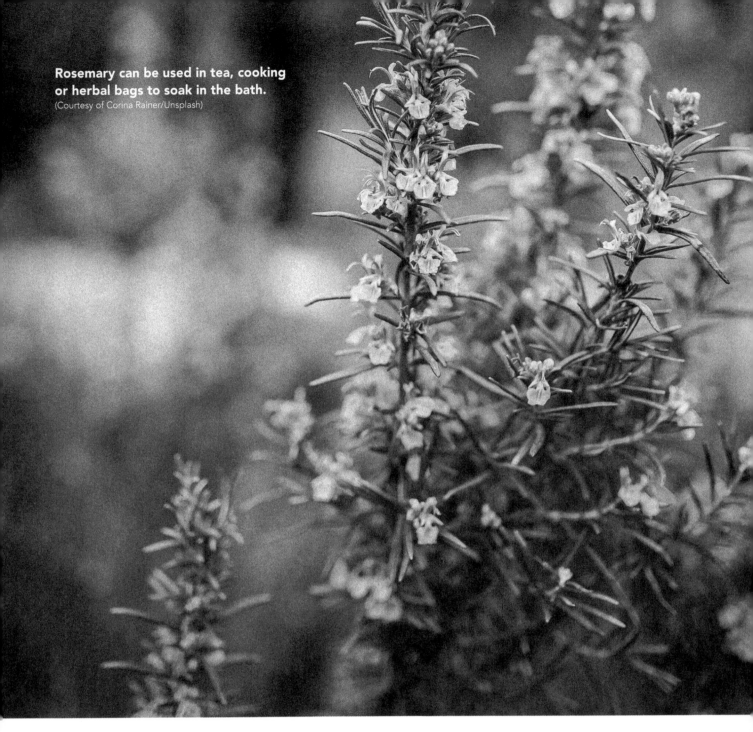

Rosemary can be used in tea, cooking or herbal bags to soak in the bath.
(Courtesy of Corina Rainer/Unsplash)

ROSEMARY (ROSMARINUS OFFICINALIS)

There's nothing nicer than the smell of rosemary in a field or roasting in the oven. It has many uses and is often included in cleaning products, deodorants and toners.

How to grow: Ideally plant rosemary outside as it can grow and spread to quite a distance. Rosemary likes to be dry, so don't overwater it. When the plant flowers, trim off the tops. These can be used in tea, cooking or herbal bags to soak in the bath.

∽ TOP TIP ∽

For a quick morning boost rub some rosemary leaves between your hands – it'll help focus your mind.

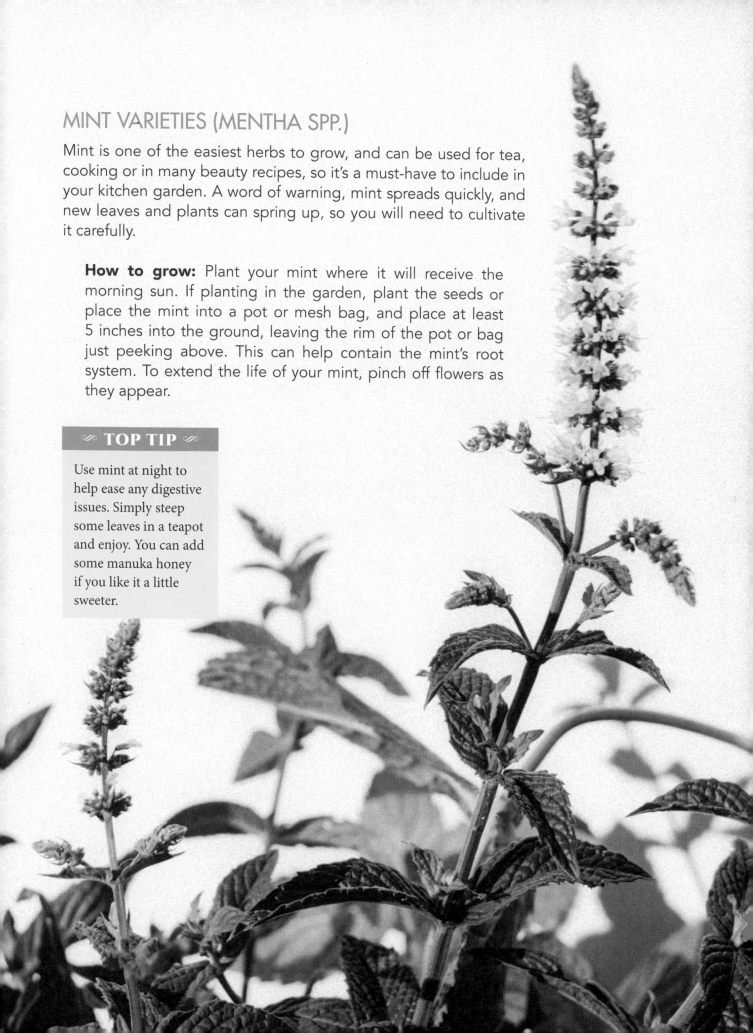

MINT VARIETIES (MENTHA SPP.)

Mint is one of the easiest herbs to grow, and can be used for tea, cooking or in many beauty recipes, so it's a must-have to include in your kitchen garden. A word of warning, mint spreads quickly, and new leaves and plants can spring up, so you will need to cultivate it carefully.

How to grow: Plant your mint where it will receive the morning sun. If planting in the garden, plant the seeds or place the mint into a pot or mesh bag, and place at least 5 inches into the ground, leaving the rim of the pot or bag just peeking above. This can help contain the mint's root system. To extend the life of your mint, pinch off flowers as they appear.

∾ TOP TIP ∾

Use mint at night to help ease any digestive issues. Simply steep some leaves in a teapot and enjoy. You can add some manuka honey if you like it a little sweeter.

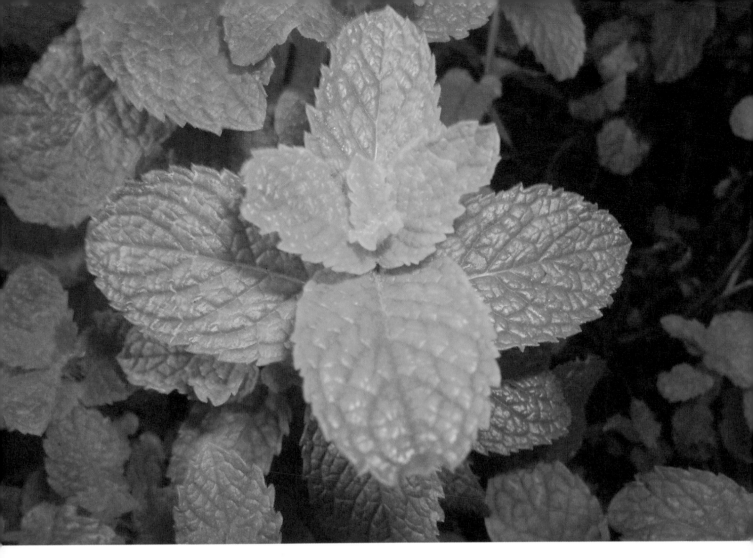

Lemon balm may help to relieve feelings of despondency and depression.
(Courtesy of Pxhere)

LEMON BALM (MELISSA OFFICINALIS)

This is an often-forgotten-about herb, although it has numerous benefits, including helping to relieve feelings of despondency and depression. It may be used to help treat and encourage healing of cold sores, and is an ideal addition to skin treatments. The herb can be used in tea and is a wonderfully comforting treat to have at night before bed.

How to grow: Lemon balm can spread and grow up to 1–3 feet high, so make sure you give it enough room. It enjoys full sun, although if you can provide the plant with some afternoon shade the leaves will less likely wilt or lose their fragrance. Once the plant is established (typically when the flowers begin to open), you can use the leaves at any time to enjoy in your tea or dried. Cut each stem just above a pair of leaves to encourage future growth.

To dry, strip the leaves from the stem. Using either a dehydrator or screen, allow to dry, keeping the leaves in a cool, dark place. One other, quicker way, is to place the leaves on metal baking trays and leave in the sun until dried.

∞ TOP TIP ∞

You'll need to infuse lemon balm flowers in order to use the oil in your beauty recipes as it's more effective this way. Follow the instructions previously given for making calendula oil.

CHAMOMILE (MATRICARIA CHAMOMILLA)

Chamomile is used in many products, including shampoo, conditioner, tea and skincare. Its healing properties help to reduce redness and calm inflamed skin. The plants produce pretty flowers, so they can be used to edge your garden for extra colour.

How to grow: Plant chamomile in a shaded area with good drainage. It thrives quite well without much attention, so you'll only need to water once every couple of weeks.

Chamomile can be used to help reduce insomnia, but is also used in many beauty products and recipes.

∾ TOP TIP ∾

You can also use chamomile tea bags to reduce the appearance of tired, puffy eyes (just make sure they're no longer hot after you've boiled them!). Make yourself a pot to help calm nerves, then use the teabags afterwards to reduce signs of strain around the eye area.

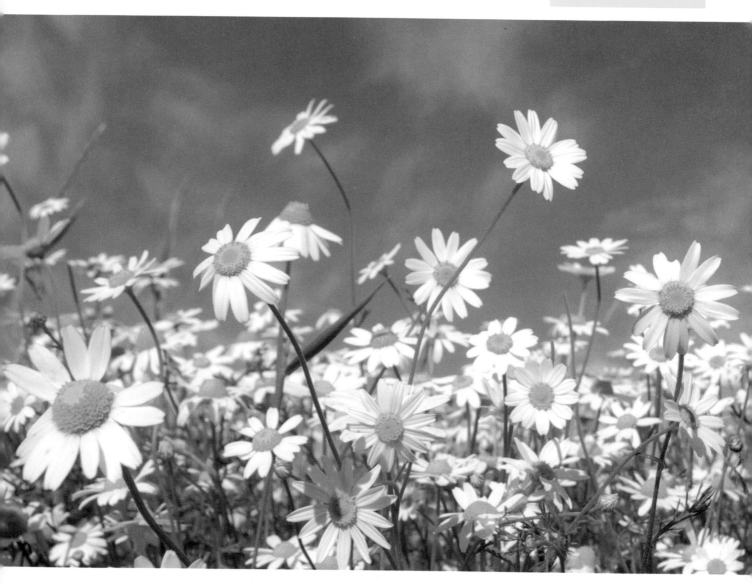

Plant some aloe vera to have on hand to treat sunburn, burns or scrapes.

ALOE VERA

Every garden, windowsill or balcony should have at least one aloe vera plant. They're simple to grow but have numerous health benefits. You can snap off a small part of the plant and squeeze out the gel-like substance to use on sunburn, dry skin, cold sores, scratches or irritated areas. And if you've accidentally burnt your skin on the oven or a baking tray, a squeeze of aloe vera oil can do wonders for reducing the pain and also speeds up the healing process. When cutting the leaf to use, cut at an angle. This will allow the leaf to seal up and continue to grow.

How to grow: You can use almost any soil to grow your aloe vera succulent. It can be grown indoors and outdoors, although as it's spiky it may be best planted outdoors if you have children. It will need drainage, so ensure the area it's planted in doesn't get too muddy or damp.

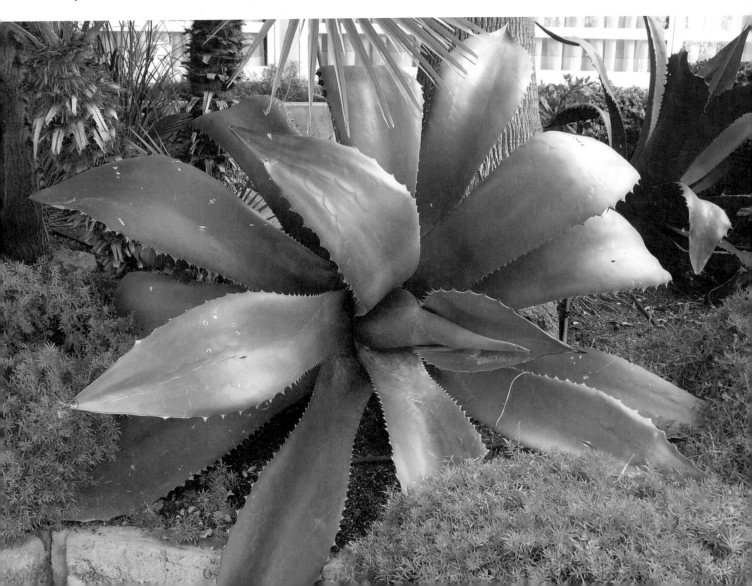

CHAPTER SIX

DIY BEAUTY –
WHAT YOU'LL NEED

AS YOU'VE NOW READ, many beauty products can cause more harm than good, particularly if used in high quantities. And this is where you come in. Making your own beauty products doesn't mean you'll need a white coat and laboratory. Many ingredients used by the large cosmetic houses can be found in your garden, pantry or on the shelf of your local health food store. And once you

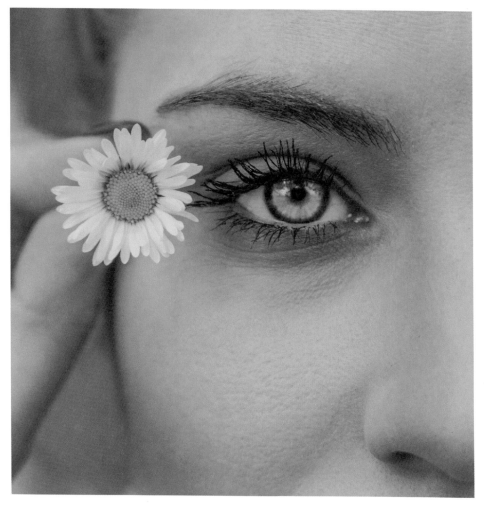

(Courtesy of Angelos Michalopoulos/Unsplash)

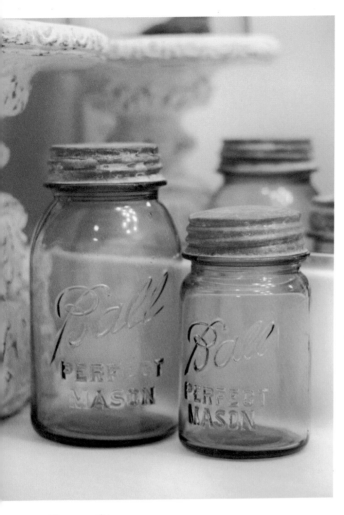

By creating your own beauty products you'll have access to your own bespoke, and specially tailored remedies to suit your skin needs.

(Jen Theodore/Unsplash)

discover the beauty of making your own lotions and potions, you'll never go back to store-bought beauty products again.

Embracing a natural beauty routine is one of the best decisions you can make for your body and overall health. Nature is filled with wonderful healing ingredients that can be used to soothe and heal.

Fruits, in particular, make excellent beauty treatments. If you look at the label of a moisturiser or exfoliant, it's likely that it will contain a 'fruit extract' in the ingredient list. Some fruits have astringent qualities, which means they'll remove dead skin painlessly and easily. This enables the skin cells underneath to breathe properly. When dead skin cells accumulate, you can be left with clogged pores, breakouts, and a dull-looking complexion. Other fruits can nurture and calm your skin, and can be used to treat acne, spots, injuries and scars.

Vegetables are an ideal skincare ingredient: they have an anti-inflammatory effect on damaged, inflamed and sensitive skin. Most vegetables contain vitamin A, which is required by the skin's top layer, the epidermis, to produce healthy cells. Masks and treatments using vegetables tend to have an immediate cooling or calming effect and are an excellent remedy for sunburn, allergic reactions, eczema or pimples.

Creating your own skincare range has many benefits: you'll save money (when you buy an over-the-counter item, you're paying for the marketing, advertising and packaging), you'll be less likely to have a reaction to hidden chemicals, you'll be able to personalise the recipe for your own skincare needs and you'll have less waste. In fact, some of the recipes in this book use leftover food and ingredients, so you'll be contributing even less to your rubbish.

And there's nothing better than pampering yourself: whether it's an afternoon spent in your garden, relaxing with a good book, or applying your luxurious skincare, these are wonderful habits to get into for a healthy mind and body. By setting aside some time every day to treat yourself, your skin, and your soul, you, and the world around you, will be a happier, healthier place.

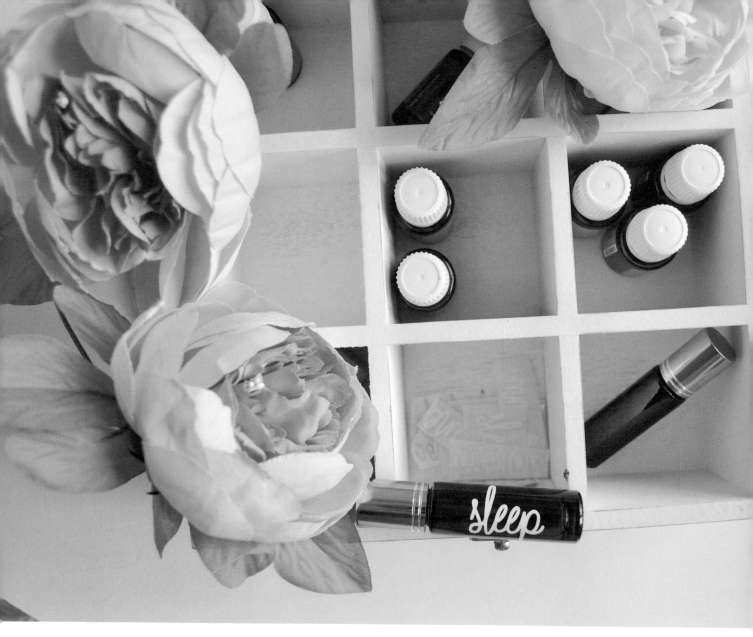

A WORD ON ESSENTIAL OILS

While many of the recipes included in this book use fruits, vegetables and herbs, it's important to note the place essential oils can play in skincare.

Essential oils have been used for centuries to treat and pamper skin. They contain anti-inflammatory, antibacterial and soothing properties and some oils can also help sooth dry, oily or acne-prone skin.

A word of warning: never apply neat essential oils directly to your skin; they always need to be diluted in either oil, water or a liquid base. It's always a good idea to test a new essential oil to ensure you don't react to it – ideally, use the inside of your wrist.

Essential oils are important part of skin care and can help treat and pamper your skin.
(Courtesy of Brittany Neale/Unsplash)

SKIN CONDITIONS – AND ESSENTIAL OILS – AT A GLANCE

Skin type		What to use
Oily	Excess oil production, shiny t-zone, large pores, blackhead and acne prone	Melon seed, sunflower, evening primrose, bergamot, rose geranium, clary sage, lemon, lavender
Sensitive	Tight (particularly after showering or washing), prone to flakiness, stinging, redness, reacts to some products	Rose hip, jojoba, calendula, olive, chamomile, rose, neroli, lavender, sandalwood
Dry	Dull, rough or flaky. Tends to be itchy	Cocoa butter, rose hip oil, jojoba, coconut, sesame, pomegranate
Normal/ combination	Shiny forehead, nose and chin, dry or normal elsewhere	Jojoba, hemp, sesame, pomegranate
Allergy prone – dermatitis and eczema	Flaking, redness, irritation (mainly hands, neck and face)	Evening primrose, rose hip, chamomile, rose
Ageing	Small or deep lines. Prone to dehydration particularly in the morning	Grape seed, apricot, rose hip, jojoba, sesame, frankincense, rose, neroli
Rosacea	Redness, clogged, bumpy skin, visible veins	Evening primrose, rose hip, chamomile, rosewood, rose geranium
Acne	Clogged pores, red lumps, painful bumps	Evening primrose, rose hip, chamomile, lavender

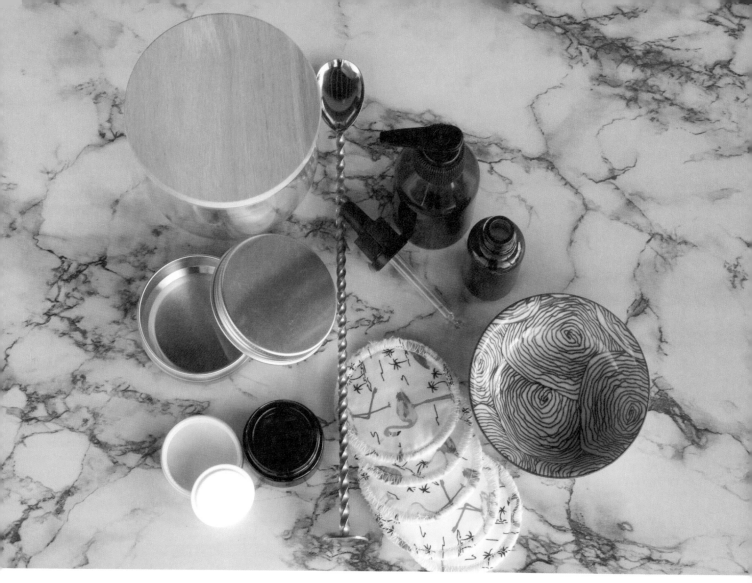

GETTING STARTED

What you'll need.
(Courtesy of Conleth Prosser)

Ready to start your own skincare range? Take a look at the shopping list (on page XX) for the cupboard and fridge staples you'll need. There's no need to spend a huge amount of money – most of the ingredients are probably already sitting in your fridge or cupboard. Some of the base oils or creams will need to be purchased, but they do last a long time.

This list may seem exhaustive and expensive, but there are plenty which you will probably already have to hand – such as bananas, yoghurt, oatmeal. Ideally, buy organic where possible. Many health food stores also sell several of the ingredients required in self-serve sizes and so you won't have to purchase a 1kg bag of oats, when you just need a couple of tablespoons! (Although this is one ingredient I recommend you always have in your cupboard.)

Equipment wise, collate the following for your concoctions. Make sure all items are spotlessly clean, dry and that all lids seal completely. This will help prevent bacteria growth, or leakages.

- Mixing bowl made of plastic or glass (metal bowls oxidise when they come into contact with fruit or vegetable juices).
- Storage jars made of plastic or glass. Your natural beauty products should be stored in your refrigerator, unless specified. Recipes containing eggs or milk should be kept no longer than six hours.
- Small containers or old lipstick tubes which are now empty (for the lip glosses).
- Cotton wool balls or a reusable facial wipe.
- Hair band (for face masks).
- Spatula – plastic or wooden is best.
- Cocktail-style long-handled spoon (to pour or scoop ingredients into bowls and containers).

NB: There are many stores now offering DIY beauty ingredients. Online, you can source hundreds of products, which also come with instructions and recipes.

Each recipe in this book will give storing suggestions to ensure that your beauty products don't spoil.

SHOPPING LIST

- Aloe vera juice
- Apple cider vinegar
- Apples
- Avocado
- Avocado oil
- Baking soda
- Bananas
- Beeswax
- Carrots
- Citrus juice (lemon, grapefruit, orange)
- Coconut oil
- Cucumber
- Essential oils (such as peppermint, eucalyptus, lavender, chamomile)
- Extra-virgin olive oil
- Heavy cream
- Honey (manuka or local honey is best)
- Lemons

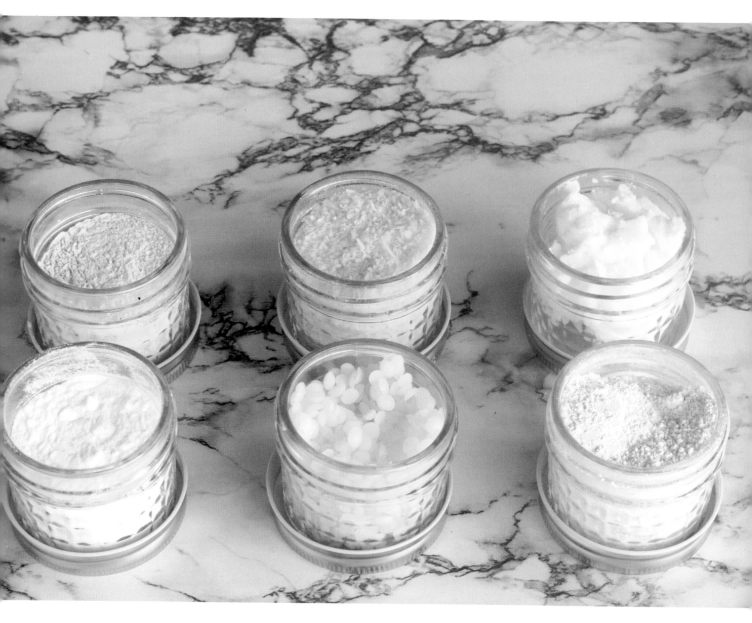

- Mangoes
- Oats
- Olive oil
- Pineapples
- Plain yoghurt
- Rose geranium oil
- Rose hip oil
- Sea salt
- Shea butter
- Vitamin E capsules (or vitamin E liquid)
- Watermelon

Most ingredients are available at your local supermarket or natural health store.

(Courtesy of Conleth Prosser)

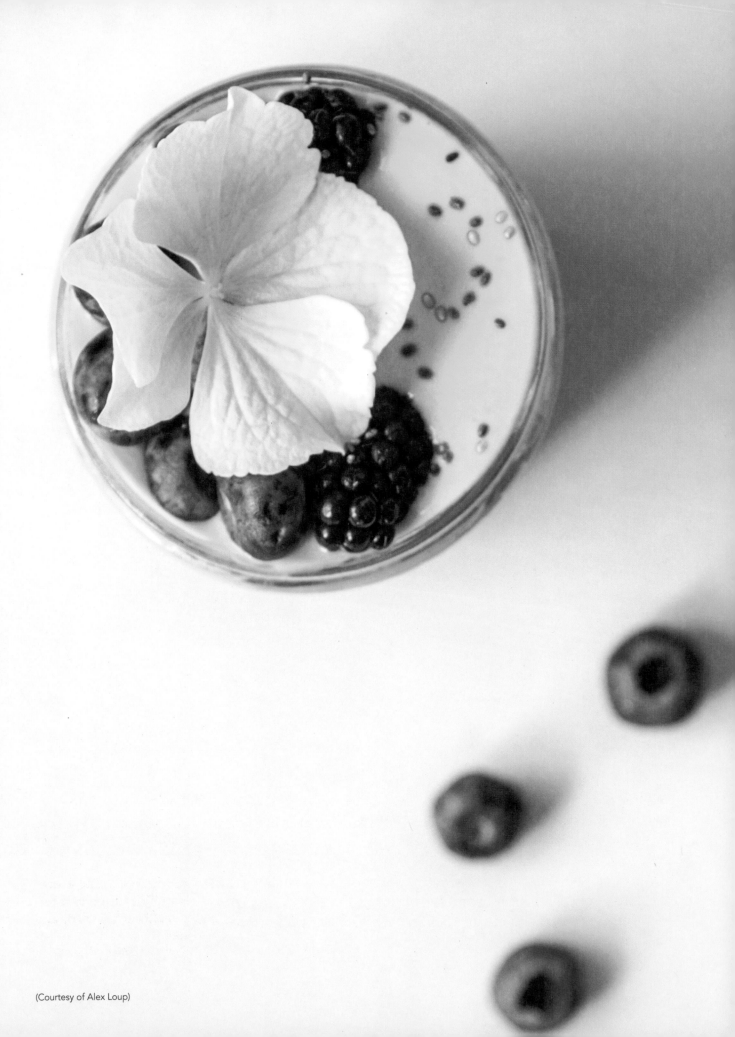

CHAPTER SEVEN

YOUR DIY BEAUTY RECIPES FOR FACE

THE FOLLOWING RECIPES have been designed for normal skin, unless otherwise specified. If you do experience, or have experienced, reactions to certain ingredients or skin products in the past take it slowly. Ideally, test the concoction on your inner arm or wrist before applying.

If a recipe is one-use only, this will be indicated; storage suggestions are made for each treatment.

Remember, beauty, and the act of treating yourself should be enjoyable. Take your time, enjoy the process as much as the application. If you're applying a mask, make an event of it, by having a bath while the ingredients do their work, or watch a favourite TV show. Relaxing and taking care of yourself is just as important as what you eat, and what you use on your skin.

So light some candles, fill the bathtub with some relaxing essential oils and grab your favourite book. Apply your treatments, lie back and allow yourself to be pampered.

CLEANSING YOUR SKIN

Removing the day's dirt, makeup and pollution is a vital step towards healthy skin. Cleansing morning and night is a must, as removing anything sitting on top of your skin will help prevent skin breakouts and allow your renewed skin cells to emerge.

To cleanse properly, use a headband or similar to pull your hair away from your face. Use lukewarm water only (never hot!) and recyclable towelling wipes or muslin cloths to remove the product. Remember not to pull or tug at your skin as this can cause premature ageing.

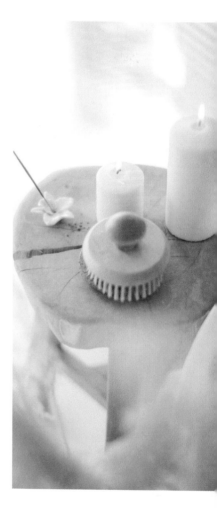

Taking time out of your busy life is important for a healthy mind, body and soul.
(Courtesy of Elly Fairytale/Pexels)

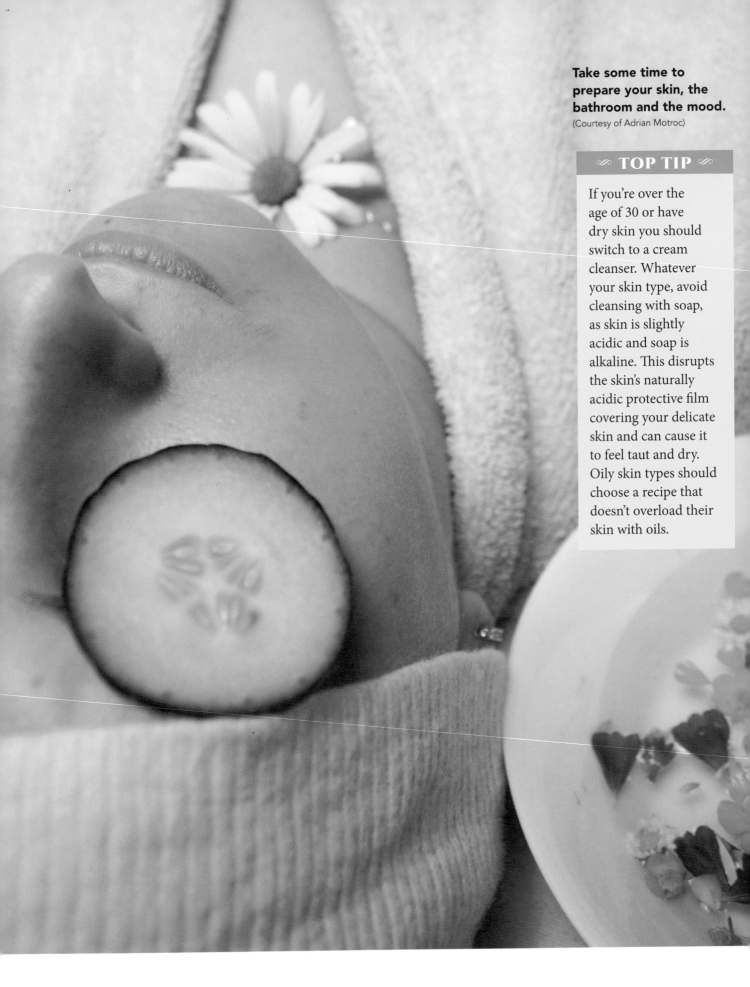

Take some time to prepare your skin, the bathroom and the mood.
(Courtesy of Adrian Motroc)

∽ TOP TIP ∽

If you're over the age of 30 or have dry skin you should switch to a cream cleanser. Whatever your skin type, avoid cleansing with soap, as skin is slightly acidic and soap is alkaline. This disrupts the skin's naturally acidic protective film covering your delicate skin and can cause it to feel taut and dry. Oily skin types should choose a recipe that doesn't overload their skin with oils.

DIY CLEANSERS

A DREAM CLEAN

It's not just good for your waistline! Lettuce is also a great way to cleanse your skin. As it contains vitamins, sulphur, silicon and phosphorous it's ideal to help naturally restore your skin's pH level (the measure of dryness) and balance out a reddened complexion. Recommended for all skin types.

Ingredients
- 1/2 head of lettuce
- 4 cups of water
- 1/8 tsp of benzoin (this is a tincture available at health food stores)

Method
Place the saucepan and water over medium heat and bring to boil. Once the water is boiling, lower the heat and add the lettuce leaves. Simmer for one hour. Remove from heat and allow to cool. Strain the liquid into an oven-proof dish. Stir in the benzoin tincture. Pour into a bottle or jar, replacing the lid tightly. Store in the fridge for up to one week.

Use the lotion to cleanse your skin in the morning or at night.

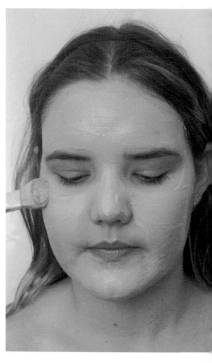

Dream clean – use a makeup brush to apply your face mask.
(Courtesy of Conleth Prosser)

TOMATO AND MILK CLEANSER

Using tomatoes on your skin is a great way to help mop up any free radical damage caused by pollution and environmental factors.

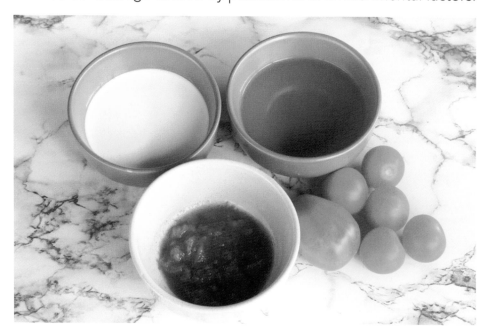

Tomatoes also have a high fruit acid content which will gently peel away dead skin.
(Courtesy of Conleth Prosser)

Tomatoes also have a high fruit acid content; combined with the lactic acid in the milk this cleansing lotion will gently peel away dead skin. This is ideal to use if your skin is flaky or you've been sunburnt recently.

Recommended for normal and oily skin types.

Ingredients
- 1 medium very ripe tomato
- Fresh whole milk
- Bottled or spring water

Method
Juice or blend the tomato until it is pure liquid. Strain the mixture through a piece of muslin. Add the tomato juice to an equal amount of fresh milk (i.e. 1 cup tomato juice to 1 cup of milk). Pour into a bottle, or spritzer and keep in the fridge no longer than five days.

This can be used twice a day – ideally leave it on for around five minutes before rinsing off to help remove dead skin cells.

TURN BACK TIME
If you're over the age of 30 or have dry skin, then a cream-based cleanser is best. You'll notice the difference immediately as your skin soaks up the excess moisture. Even if your skin is oily, don't shy away from creamy moisturisers. According to skin guru Zoe Foster Blake, oil attracts oil, so using oil-based cleansers will actually removes the excess slick, not adds to it.

Ingredients
- 1 tbsp thick dairy cream (chilled from the fridge)
- 2 drops rose essential oil

Method
Mix the essential oil into the cream until combined. Store in an airtight container in the fridge for up to three days.

Combine and use as you would your usual cleanser. Massage well, firmly pressing the lotion into your skin in an upward motion. (Tip: begin cleansing at your chest area and work your way upwards. This helps to promote good circulation.) Remove with a damp cloth or wipe, following with a splash of cool water.

GREAT OATS
This cleanser gently removes excess oils, makeup and dirt without stripping the skin of its natural oils. Oats are excellent cleansers, of

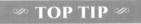
✺ TOP TIP ✺
For extra fragrance and calm, add a couple of drops of calming and nourishing essential oil. I love rose oil or lavender, but choose whatever you have available, or prefer.

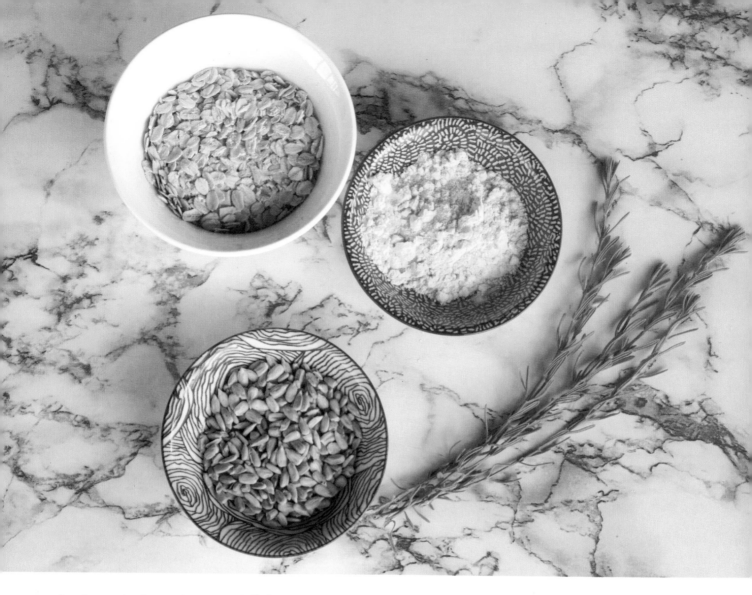

both topical products and flaky skin. The slight roughness of the oats will gently exfoliate dead skin cells but is gentle enough to do so without irritating sensitive skin. Sunflower seeds contain oils which add moisture to your skin.

Oats make excellent cleansers and exfoliators and can be used on the face and body.

(Courtesy of Conleth Prosser)

Ingredients
- 1/2 cup ground oats
- 1/3 cup finely ground sunflower seeds
- 1/4 cup finely ground almond meal
- 1 drop lavender essential oil
- Water

Method
Mix the dry ingredients together in a bowl until a thick paste is formed. Scoop out the mixture into your hand and apply to damp skin (make sure you cleanse your neck, chest and face). If the mixture feels too dry, add some water to dilute it. Store in an airtight container in the fridge for up to six months.

GENTLE EXFOLIATING CLEANSER

Not just for drinking, apple cider vinegar (ACV) is often used as a great cleanser to help exfoliate dead skin cells. This is due to the malic acid (similar to alpha-hydroxy acid), which rids your skin of flaky skin and may even help even out an uneven complexion. I find that it works well on menopausal or perimenopausal reddened skin. Use just once or twice a week, alternating with a gentle toner so that you don't overburden your skin.

Ingredients

It's important to dilute ACV as it can be irritating for all skin types, not just sensitive skin. Match like for like, whatever amount you decide to use.

- 100ml water
- 100ml ACV

Method

Combine in an amber bottle and shake well. Only make enough to last you for a week. Store in the refrigerator and apply on a facial wipe or spritz onto the skin. Allow it to settle on the skin for five to ten minutes, before removing it with warm water. Follow with serum and moisturiser.

OIL BE THERE FOR YOU CLEANSER

One of my favourite suppliers of DIY beauty ingredients is an Australian-based company called Biome (biome.com.au). They have kindly shared their DIY oil cleanser recipe with you. This oil cleanser works to clean, heal and hydrate your skin. Use it every day to help heal acne, dryness or combination skin. When massaged into the skin, oils in the cleanser bind to surface impurities and pull out the impurities without clogging pores. The impurities can be rinsed away and the skin is left feeling clean, soft and hydrated.

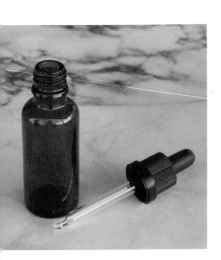

Use a pipette to measure out your ingredients and dosages.
(Courtesy Conleth Prosser)

Ingredients

- 1 tbsp castor oil
- 1 tbsp jojoba oil
- 2 tbsp apricot kernel oil
- 2 tbsp hemp seed oil
- Essential oils if desired – use 1 drop each of the following: lavender, frankincense, patchouli and ylang ylang
- Amber dropper bottle 50ml
- Store out of sunlight and use within six months.

Method

Place oils (and essential oils if desired) into your chosen dropper bottle and shake well. Leave to infuse overnight. To use, shake the bottle well. Splash warm water on your face to open up the pores. Using your fingers, gently massage 3–5 drops of the oil mixture into your face, using a circular motion for about a minute. This will loosen the dirt from your pores and help draw it to the surface. With a warm, wet washcloth, dab your face by pressing lightly all over, allowing the oils to penetrate deeper. Rinse the washcloth with hot water and place flat onto your face to steam. Afterwards, thoroughly wipe your face with the cloth. Rinse again and repeat if necessary to ensure all the oil is removed. Splash your face with cold water to close pores. Your skin will feel soft, smooth and highly moisturised.

CLEANSING TREATMENT

STRAWBERRY STEAM

If you feel that your skin needs a little extra TLC when doing a cleanse/steam, then this is a wonderful one for all skin types. The herbs in this recipe help to soothe and rebalance problematic skin, adding natural oils and calming any irritation and redness.

Ingredients
- 1 tbsp dried lavender (or 1 drop lavender oil)
- ½ litre boiled water (now slightly cooled)
- ½ cup fresh strawberries

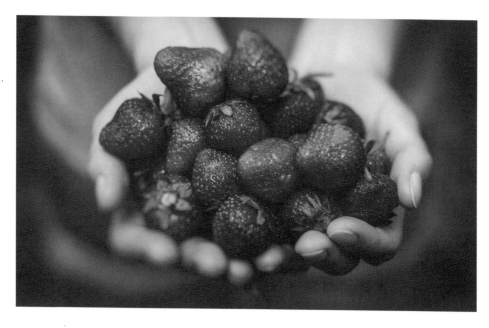

Strawberries are a wonderful way to soothe and rebalance troubled skin.
(Courtesy of Artur Rutkowski)

Method (you'll need a large towel for this)

Pour the boiled water into an oven- or microwave-proof bowl. Add the lavender oil and strawberries. Allow the heat to absorb the oil and the scent of the berries. Place your face over the steam and cover your head with a towel. Leave for 5–15 minutes (although you may need to take regular breaks and stop if it feels too hot). Rise your face with cool water and pat dry.

ROSE AND CHAMOMILE STEAM

Rose has a wonderful scent which helps you to relax. Paired with the calming properties of chamomile, this is a great steam to use post-cleanser, and pre-mask treatment. Remember not to place your face too close to the hot water – around 10cm away is ideal.

Ingredients
- 1 litre boiling water
- Pinch of rose petals (or rose oil)
- Pinch of chamomile flowers (or chamomile tea bags/chamomile oil)

Rose brings with it a gorgeous scent to help you relax. (Courtesy of Pexels)

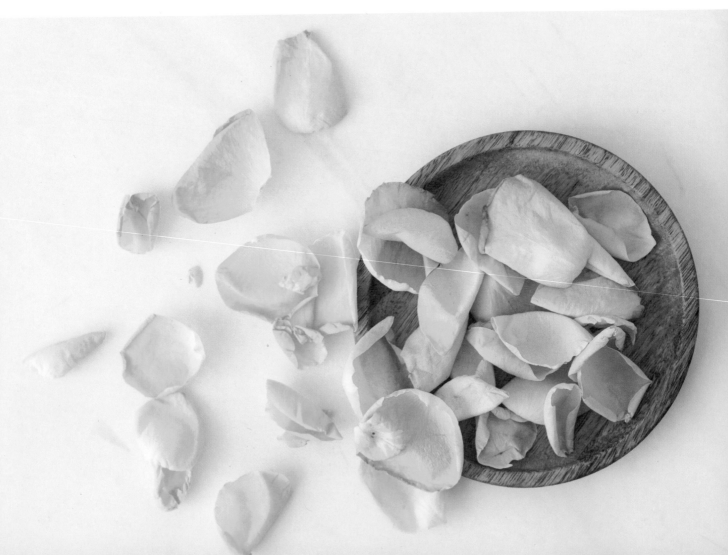

Method

Pour the boiling water into a bowl, followed by the rose and chamomile. Allow to steep and the water to slightly cool, before placing your face over the steam with a towel over your head. Steam for around five minutes.

EUCALYPTUS FACIAL STEAM

Calming for reddened skin, this steam is also ideal if your skin is congested or you are suffering from seasonal allergies.

Ingredients
- 1 litre boiling water
- 3–5 drops eucalyptus essential oil

Method

Pour the boiling water into a bowl and add the eucalyptus oil drops. Cover your head with a towel and place your face over the pan, Breathe in through your nose and out through your mouth for around five minutes. Apply a soothing moisturiser or face mask afterwards to continue the treatment.

Toners

Toners rehydrate, cool, nourish and refresh your skin. They remove any remaining traces of dirt, makeup or oil your cleanser may have not removed, along with any dead skin cells. There is mixed thought over whether toners are a necessary part of the cleansing regime – many people instead double cleanse to feel properly clean. I like the cooling astringent properties of a toner. If you do too, but don't want to use one, consider making a spritzer instead. This will plump your skin out and provide a dewy base for your moisturiser. (See page XX for recipes).

COOL AS A CUCUMBER

Use cucumber to soothe irritated skin, as it contains calming astringents, which reduce puffiness and redness. Chamomile is also an excellent soothing ingredient – ideal if your skin is super sensitive. As cucumber is so gentle on the skin, this toner can be used every day. Ideal for sensitive skin.

Ingredients
- 1 cucumber
- ½ carrot (juiced)

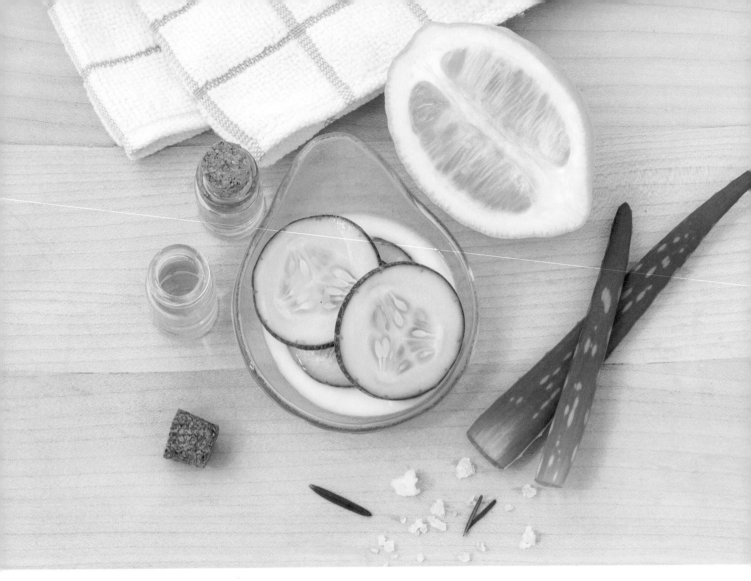

Be cool as a cucumber with this calming toner.
(Courtesy of Conleth Prosser)

- ¼ cup chamomile tea (cooled)
- ½ cup lemon juice

Method
Juice the cucumber and carrot. Add chamomile tea and lemon juice and combine well in a glass jar. Use a cotton wool ball to apply to your face. Keep refrigerated and store for no longer than three days.

HERBAL TONER
This sweet smelling toner is suitable for all skin types. The grapefruit seed extract will help to eradicate any dry, flaky skin as it contains AHAs which dissolve dead skin cells. Rose water helps to calm any irritation and is a great ingredient to have to hand.

Ingredients
- 125ml rose water
- 1 tsp vegetable glycerine

- 1 tsp pressed organic almond oil
- 12 drops grapefruit seed extract

Method
Combine all ingredients in a jar and shake well to blend. Apply to skin and massage, beginning at your jawline, working upwards. Leave for sixty seconds and rinse with lukewarm water. Will keep refrigerated for around a month.

GREEN PEACE TONER
Rich in anti-oxidants, this toner may help fight the ageing process as it protects the epidermis from external factors such as sunlight, pollution and smoke. Combined with mint, which adds a refreshing quality to the toner, this treatment should be used by those with normal or combination skin. Use daily, followed by your moisturiser.

Ingredients
- 200ml mineral water
- 4 tsp green tea leaves
- 1 tsp mint leaves
- 1 tsp lemon juice

Make the most of your herb garden and use them in your toners, bath or tea.
(Courtesy of Conleth Prosser)

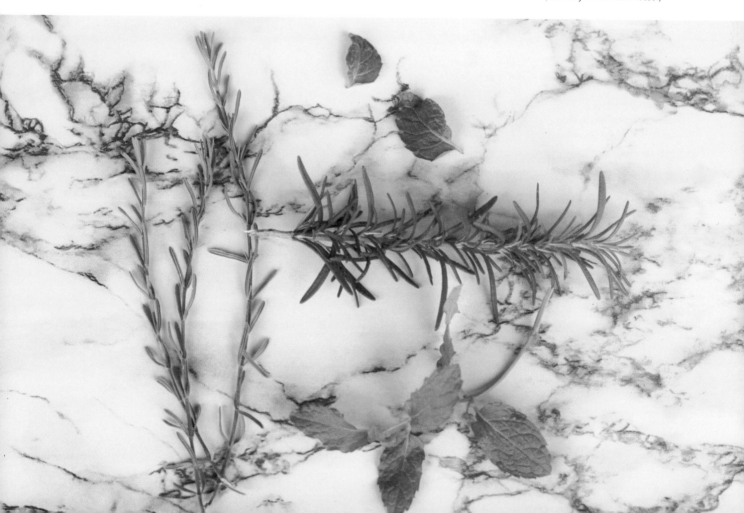

Method

Make an infusion with the leaves in a tea pot and add the lemon juice. Strain and allow the liquid to cool. Pour into a spritzer bottle for easy use. Keep in the refrigerator for no longer than seven days.

CELERY TONER

As per the recommendation for celery as a mask, this green vegetable can also be used as a toner and is a great detoxifying drink (albeit a bitter one). The ingredients used in this toner help to protect your skin and cool it down, especially if it's feeling wind- or sun-burnt.

Ingredients
- 3 tomatoes, seeded and halved
- 4 lettuce leaves
- 5 celery stems
- ½ cup diced carrots
- ¼ cup basil leaves
- ¼ cup cucumber juice

Method

Put all the ingredients into a blender, along with two cups of water. Pour the juice into a spray bottle, either adding ice, or placing into the fridge to cool. Spray the liquid over your face, followed with a facial wipe or muslin cloth. Wash with cool water and pat dry. Keep in the fridge for no longer than five days.

MOISTURISERS

Applying moisturiser day and night is a must to help keep your skin hydrated and smooth. A good moisturiser should keep your skin feeling soft and smooth all day long – if your skin begins to feel taut or dry after a few hours, you may need a cream-based or thicker lotion.

SERUM RECIPE

Most commercial serums are expensive – understandably, as a good serum helps to reduce the appearance of age spots, softens fine lines and reduces irritations and redness. However, most basic serums have similar ingredients to the recipe below. One advantage of making your own is choosing which essential oil you prefer. (The

☙ **TOP TIP** ☙

Applying a serum is a great base for your moisturiser. It will help trap moisturiser and you won't need to apply as much of your DIY cream – yet you'll achieve the same, if not better, results.

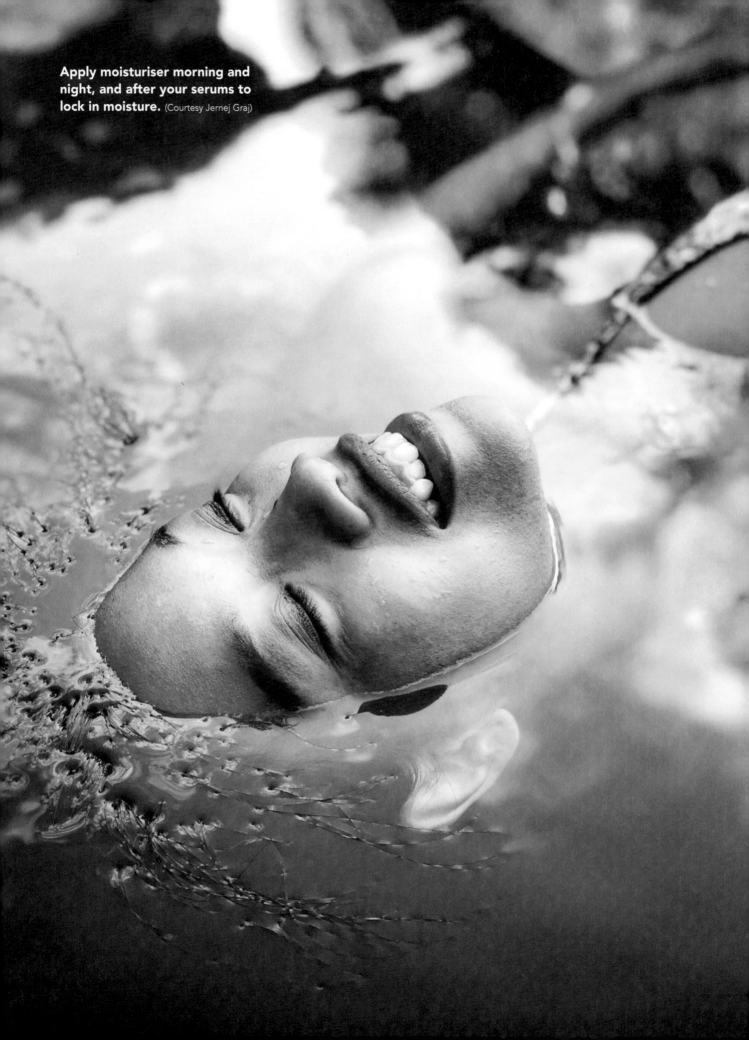

Apply moisturiser morning and night, and after your serums to lock in moisture. (Courtesy Jernej Graj)

essential oil guide on page XX will help you decide which is best for your skin type)

SIMPLY SMOOTH SERUM

This is a wonderfully scented serum for any skin type. Use morning and night.

Ingredients
- 2 tbsp shea oil
- 2 tbsp jojoba oil
- 20 drops essential oil of your choice (I like rose, frankincense and geranium. Geranium is particularly good for more mature, drier skin)
- 50ml amber glass dropper bottle

Method
Combine all ingredients into the glass bottle. Shake well to combine. Use 3–5 drops morning and night, after cleansing and before moisturising. I like to use a couple of drops around the mouth and eye area throughout the day if my skin is feeling taut or dry. Store away from sunlight. This should keep for as long as needed.

EVERYDAY MOISTURISER

Moisturiser protects your skin from the elements and helps to keep moisture trapped into your skin cells. Throughout the day air conditioning, glare from screens, contact with phone and hands means that we're regularly putting a lot of stress on our skin. A good moisturiser helps to protect your skin from these external elements.

Note: As none of these moisturisers contain SPF you should apply your sunscreen after your serum and moisturiser. Ideally, use a foundation or powder with an SPF on top of your daily cream.

Ingredients
- 150ml almond oil
- 90g cocoa butter
- 30g beeswax
- 125ml distilled water
- 1 tsp royal jelly
- 30 drops grapefruit seed extract oil

Method
Combine the oils, cocoa butter and beeswax melting them over a low heat. Stir the ingredients together slowly, keeping an eye on

the bottom of the pan to ensure the mixture doesn't burn or stick. Remove from the stove and add water. Blend until the mixture is thick and creamy. Add the grapefruit oils. Store in glass jars with screw-on tops. This mixture lasts around four months (discard if you notice any discolouration or mould).

THIRSTY SKIN MOISTURISER

Heating, air conditioning, lack of water and over-zealous exfoliating can all add up to dry, parched skin. Using avocado is ideal as it contains the essential fatty oils needed to replicate cells and produce collagen. Combined with the nourishing wheatgerm oil, cocoa butter and beeswax, this is an ideal moisture-replenisher for dry, tired complexions. Add an essential oil for extra scent and healing if required.

Ingredients
- 4 tbsp avocado oil
- 4 tsp wheatgerm oil

Dry skin needs extra TLC alongside a diet rich in healthy fats.
(Courtesy of Lisa Fotios)

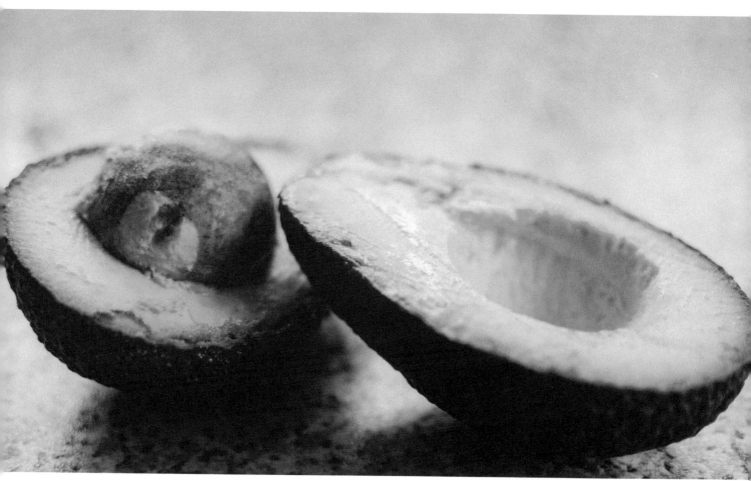

TOP TIP

If you can't be bothered making up a moisturiser, you can cheat a little. Use pure shea oil directly to the skin – it's great for dry areas such as cheeks, forehead, elbows, knees or feet. Shea oil is a lightweight version of shea butter – providing lovely rich cream to thirsty skin. Keep in your bathroom cupboard as the oil likes to remain in room temperature conditions.

TOP TIP

Shea oil can also be used as a daily conditioning treatment or add to your bath for a soothing soak.

- 25g cocoa butter
- 1 tsp beeswax
- 2 tbsp rosewater
- 10 drops geranium essential oil
- 5 drops frankincense essential oil
- 5 drops sandalwood essential oil

Method
Combine the wheatgerm and avocado oil in a heat-resistant bowl and place in a saucepan which has been half-filled with water. Heat, adding the cocao butter and beeswax until the mixture has blended. Add rosewater. Remove from the heat and add the essential oils. Allow to cool before storing in an air-tight container. Keep in the refrigerator for longevity and discard after one month.

Good for: Dry, combination, sensitive and mature skin.

SMOOTH IT OVER FACE MOISTURISER
Shea butter is wonderfully soothing and smoothing. Alongside these essential oils, all of which help to restore moisture and calm the skin, and this is a must-have product to make and use every day.

Ingredients
- $1/3$ cup shea butter
- $1/8$ cup beeswax (or ampules)
- $1/4$ cup jojoba or rose hip oil
- $1/3$ cup rose water
- $1/2$ cup aloe gel
- 15 drops frankincense essential oil
- 15 drops rose essential oil

Method
Melt the shea butter and beeswax together. While the butter and beeswax are cooling, add jojoba (or rose hip), rose water and aloe gel in a measuring jug. Warm for around one minute in a microwave. Pour the oils into the shea butter and beeswax. Use a hand mixer to blend them completely and until the mixture becomes milky and fluffy. Using a spoon or spatula, scoop out the mixture into a sealable jar. These can be stored in the fridge for up to one year.

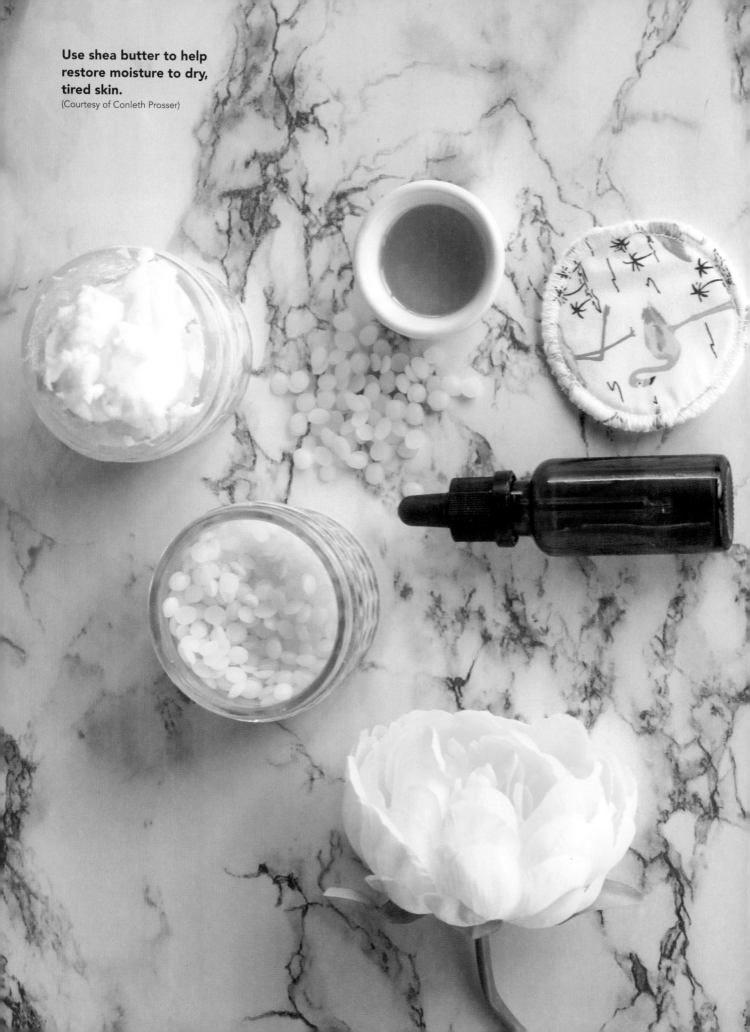

Use shea butter to help restore moisture to dry, tired skin.
(Courtesy of Conleth Prosser)

FACIAL EXFOLIANTS

Oh, sugar sugar

While eating sugar or a high sugar diet isn't great for your skin, it does have its uses in your DIY beauty recipes. The tiny granules dissolve in a cream and on your skin, gently lifting away dead skin cells, and leaving a thin, soft body scrub. You will need to follow this exfoliant with a cream cleanser to remove any residue.

Ingredients

- 250g white sugar
- 250g vegetable glycerine or avocado oil
- 2 tsp aloe vera gel
- 2 drops lavender oil
- 2 drops orange oil

Method

Mix the sugar and oils into a bowl until combined. You should be able to see and feel the sugary granules. Place a small amount into your hand. Apply to your body, scrubbing gently as you apply. Leave for one minute – you'll feel a slight tightening effect. Rinse with lukewarm water and apply moisturiser after drying. Discard any leftovers.

FACE MASKS

Is there anything better than a hot bath, candles, face mask and a glass of wine? Face masks aren't indulgent, they're a necessary part of your beauty regime. Not only will you be putting concentrated levels of ingredients into your skin, but you'll be relaxing at the same time. The heat and steam from the bath will work wonders on your stress levels and will also encourage your skin to respond positively to the treatment (by opening the pores and relaxing any stress and frown lines). Reducing stress is a vital part of your health and beauty regime, so take the time and make the space to enjoy a face mask and body treatment at least once a week.

COVER UP

Egg and lemon make an excellent purifying and skin-tightening mask. The lactic acid found in lemon aids healing with problem skin, such as spots. Egg whites are often used in face masks due to their tightening effects. Egg white contains protein, which is believed to help absorb excess oil and smooth the appearance of your skin.

Ideal for normal or oily skin.

Ingredients
- White from 1 large egg
- Juice of 1 lemon

Method

Mix the egg white and lemon juice in a bowl. Whisk until frothy. Apply a thin layer to a cleansed face – use a cotton wool pad for ease. Leave for ten minutes before removing with lukewarm water. Discard any leftovers.

WHAT A MELON MASK

Watermelon is extremely refreshing, and, as it is high in water content, it's very hydrating for the skin. This recipe is excellent for oily skin. If you have dry skin, add a banana instead of the yoghurt (or half and half) as bananas are a great way to nourish the skin.

Ingredients
- 1 cup watermelon
- 3 tbsp yoghurt

Method

Mash the watermelon in a small bowl until smooth. Add yoghurt and blend. Apply to your face and neck and cover your face with a moist facecloth. Leave for ten minutes and rinse with lukewarm water. Rinse dry. You can keep this for up to one week in an airtight container.

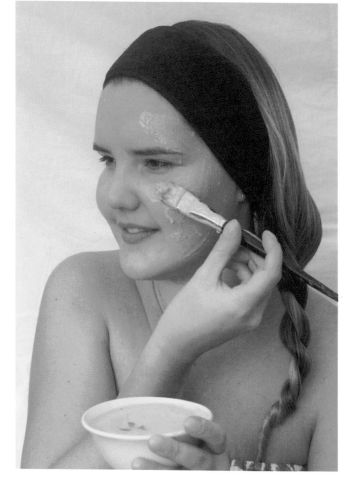

Watermelon is a great way to increase the water content of your skin. (Courtesy of Conleth Prosser)

SUMMER SMOOTH MANGO MASK

If you have a skin breakout, or pimples have left your face feeling sore and tender, this is a great way to restore some healing. Mango contains beta carotene, vitamin C and natural fruit acids – all which help to delicately slough away dead skin cells. The honey acts as a healing agent – choose local honey when you can get it.

Ingredients
- 4 tbsp chopped mango
- 1–2 tsp honey
- 1½ tsp almond oil

Method

Combine all ingredients in a bowl until relatively smooth. Apply to a cleansed face, leaving it for 15–20 minutes. Rinse off with lukewarm water, followed by a serum and your usual moisturiser. Discard any leftovers.

GO BANANAS DRY SKIN MASK

Bananas are one of the most nourishing fruits because they contain large quantities of magnesium, potassium, iron, zinc, iodine and vitamins A, B, and E. They're ideal for mature skin, helping to restore vitality and moisture.

Ingredients
- 1 banana mashed
- 1 tsp rosewater
- 2 drops glycerine

Method

Combine all ingredients in a bowl before pouring into an airtight jar. Store in the fridge and use within a week. Apply over your entire face, neck and chest for around 20–30 minutes. Remove with lukewarm water. Discard anything you don't use.

ALLURING APRICOT MASK

Apricots help your skin reset its pH balance. Combined with yoghurt which restores moisture and firms up skin, this is a great mask to apply before a night out.

Ingredients
- 1 cup dried apricots

• 2 tbsp milk powder or yoghurt

Method

Soak one cup dried apricots in hot water until they're soft and floppy. Puree in blender or food processor with two tablespoons milk powder or yoghurt. Scoop the mixture onto your face, neck and chest and allow it to set for around fifteen minutes. Remove with a damp cloth. Discard leftovers.

TOTALLY SIMPLE FACE MASK

Every cupboard has a container of baking soda – mainly because of its myriad of uses. In a face mask, baking soda helps to dissolve blackheads. The beauty of this recipe is that you can make just a small amount and apply where needed.

Ingredients
• 1 tbsp baking soda
• 2 tbsp water

Method

Mix ingredients together to create a thick paste. Apply to the chosen area and leave it for five or so minutes. Gentle remove by rubbing the baking soda into the skin, finishing off with a splash of warm water. Apply serum or diluted tea tree oil to clear the area of any bacteria. Discard leftovers.

FACE THE DAY MASK

Pineapples contain enzymes which not only exfoliate dry, flaky skin, but also promote healing. You could also use papaya if you prefer.

Ingredients
• 1 slice ripe pineapple

Method

Massage the fruit or juice onto your face. Allow to dry for about ten minutes. Rinse with lukewarm water and pat dry. Apply your usual moisturiser for soft and smooth skin. Discard after use.

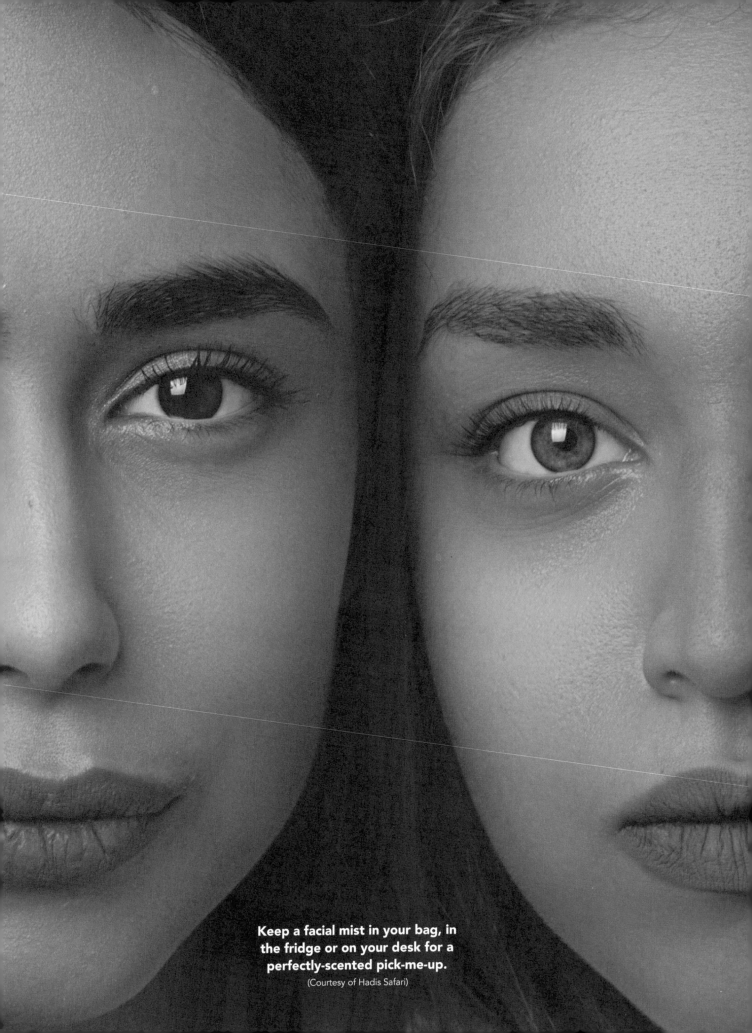

Keep a facial mist in your bag, in the fridge or on your desk for a perfectly-scented pick-me-up.

(Courtesy of Hadis Safari)

FACIAL MISTS

These refreshing sprays can be used at any time throughout the day. I like to use them before applying serum, and during the day when I'm at my computer. Spritz bottles are easily found in your chemist or supermarket (usually in the travel aisle).

WATERMELON FACIAL MIST

According to *Vogue*, watermelons are Korea's favourite fruit to use in beauty ingredients. This is a great way to use up leftover rind.

Ingredients
- Rind of ¼ watermelon chilled
- Filtered water

Method
Grate the rind and strain through a kitchen sieve or cheesecloth. Allow the liquid to gather in a bowl and add filtered water to the mix. Pour into a bottle with spritzer attachment. Store in the refrigerator and use when your skin is hot and in need of a cool drink. Discard after three weeks.

SLEEP TIGHT FACIAL MIST

Ingredients
- ½ cup water
- Lavender

Method
Fill your spritzer to the three-quarter mark. Add a few drops of lavender (you can choose the amount of scent you desire) and shake well. Store in a cool place, out of sunlight.

ROSY CHEEKS FACIAL MIST

Ingredients
- Water
- Rose oil or rosewater
- Evening Primrose oil

Method
Mix the ingredients together – using around half a spritzer bottle for the water. If you're using rosewater, aim for half and half measurements. Shake well and mist over your face. This should keep well if you store it out of direct sunlight.

GET UP AND GO FACIAL MIST

Spending time in air-conditioned spaces (or heated ones), in front of computer screens can dry out your skin, leading to frown lines and premature ageing. Even light from our devices (smart phones and tablets) can cause oxidative damage. This dry, tight feeling you may experience, can add to feelings of exhaustion and tiredness. Boost your energy levels and replenish moisture with a few sprays of this mist.

Ingredients
- Aloe vera (squeeze from your plant or a couple of drops from aloe vera juice)
- Coconut water
- 1 tbsp sweet almond oil
- 1 tbsp macadamia oil

Method

Mix all ingredients together – you can add water to dilute this further, depending on your sensitivity. There's no direction for coconut water – it depends on the size of your spritzer. This should keep for up to six months.

Every garden should have an aloe vera plant to help treat burns, dry skin, irritations and sunburn.
(Courtesy of Devon Rockola)

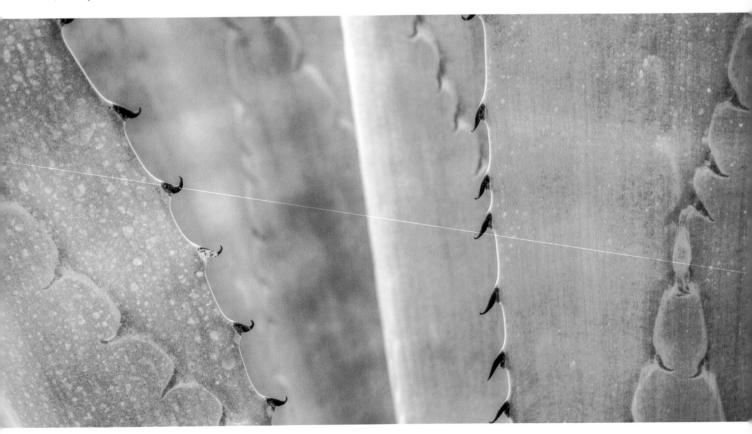

CHAPTER EIGHT

YOUR DIY BEAUTY RECIPES FOR BODY

IF YOU'RE LIKE me, I constantly forget to use moisturiser on my body – in a rush every morning, I tend to focus only on my face. Consequently my legs, arms and hands are usually crying out for some moisture. I prefer an oil-based cream for dry skin – the thicker cream recipes are lovely used at night, especially with some sleep-inducing essential oils added. Ideally, you should use a body cream directly after bathing or showering. Fill up a smaller bottle and keep in your bag to apply to your hands throughout the day.

BODY CREAMS

TOP TO TOE BODY CREAM

Essential oils can hydrate extremely dry skin and help restore its natural moisture level. The herb chamomile soothes and calms tired, sensitive skin, so this is good for sunburnt or dry skin. Rosemary and neroli are stimulating and ideal for the body as they also help to relax muscle tension. Use stimulating oils in the morning and soothing ones at night to help aid sleep.

Ingredients
- 10 drops carrot seed oil
- 60g almond, olive or sesame oil
- 10 drops lavender
- 10 drops Roman chamomile oil
OR
- 10 drops neroli oil
- 10 drops rosemary oil

Method
Apply the oil once a day after bathing or showing while your skin is

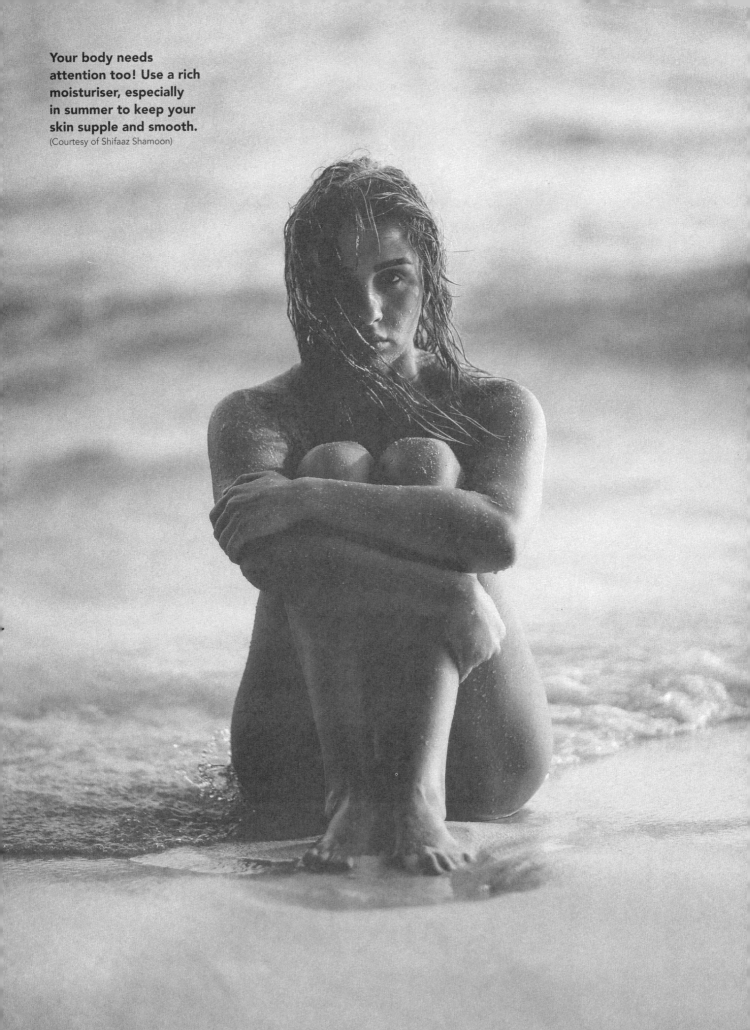

Your body needs attention too! Use a rich moisturiser, especially in summer to keep your skin supple and smooth.
(Courtesy of Shifaaz Shamoon)

still damp. This helps your body retain the moisture from bathing, as oil works as a sealant, keeping your skin hydrated and smooth. Store in an air-tight jar for no longer than four weeks.

DREAM CREAM

This recipe is based on Lush's famous sleep time body moisturiser. Apply at night, particularly to your feet, back of the knees and inner elbows. A good tip is to use a new spoon every time you scoop some of the product out – oil-based recipes will spoil if water gets into the product.

Ingredients
- 2 tbsp cocoa butter
- 8 tbsp olive oil
- 1 drop vitamin E oil (or spear a vitamin E capsule and squeeze the contents into the mixture)
- Essential oils as preferred

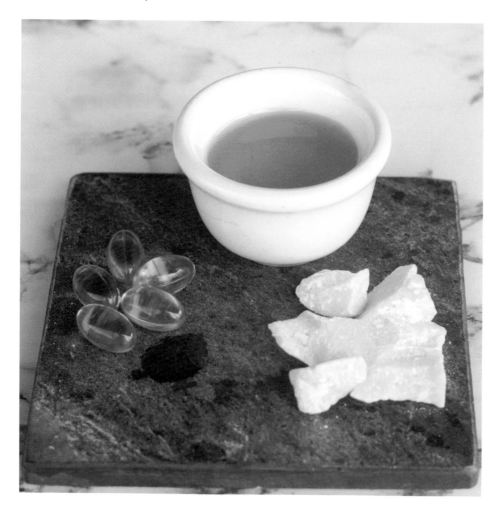

Vitamin E and cocoa butter are your two secret weapons against dry skin.
(Courtesy of Conleth Prosser)

Method

Melt the cocoa butter on a low setting. Remove from heat and add the olive oil, stirring well. Allow to cool slightly, before pouring the mixture into an ovenproof bowl. Allow to set until it's a thick cream. Add vitamin oil and whichever essential oils you've chosen. Whisk ingredients together until the mixture become light and fluffy. Scoop into an airtight container for up to three weeks.

COCOA BUTTER CREAM

If you have dry, scaly skin, or you're pregnant, or are dealing with stretch marks, cocoa butter is your go-to. Extracted from cocoa beans, it's an excellent skin softening treatment, which provides the skin with a protective barrier. It's high in antioxidants, vitamin E and healthy fatty acids. It does have a strong smell, so add a counter essential oil for added sweetness.

Ingredients

- 125g cocoa butter grated (available from specialised health food stores)
- 1 tsp almond oil
- 1 tsp light sesame oil
- 1 tsp vitamin E oil

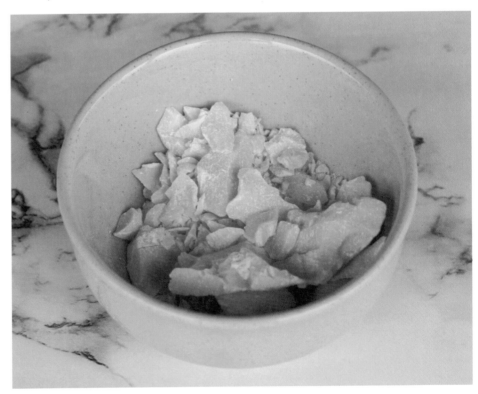

Cocoa butter can help you avoid stretch marks.
(Courtesy of Conleth Prosser)

Method

Place all the ingredients in an ovenproof glass container and heat in the microwave (around 3 mins), or in a saucepan on top of a medium stove heat. Melt and combine all the oils. Pour into a clean, air-tight container, and leave to cool. Stir for a final combination of the oils. Store in a cool, dry place. Discard after one month.

Body Exfoliants

If your skin is looking or feeling dry, scaly or just overburdened by products, a good body scrub will do wonders for revealing the glowing, smooth skin underneath. Exfoliating every few days will ensure that the creams you do use will soak into your skin and be more effective.

STRAWBERRIES FEELS FOREVER

This easy-to-make body scrub is ideal for oily skin – it's loaded with vitamin C and the acidic nature of strawberries remove any dead skin.

Ingredients

1 cup white granulated sugar
1/2 cup coconut oil
1/2 cup frozen strawberries (slightly thawed)

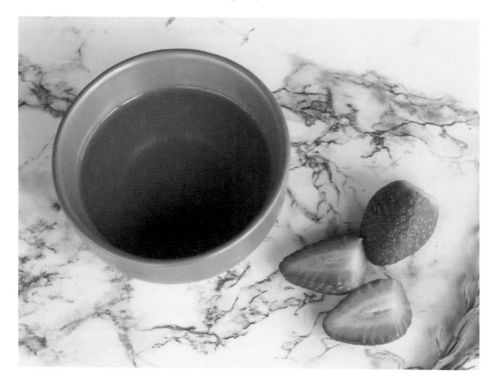

An easy-to-make body scrub which leaves your skin silky smooth.
(Courtesy of Conleth Prosser)

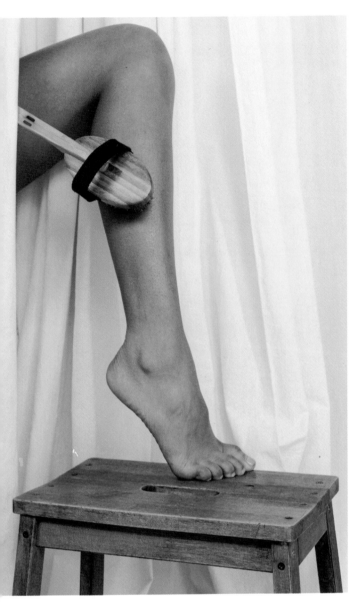

Method

Puree the strawberries in a blender — they'll resemble pink crushed ice. Melt the coconut oil in a saucepan placed on a medium heat. When the coconut oil is liquid and clear, add the sugar followed by the blended strawberries. Decant into an airtight container. This will keep in the fridge for up to one month.

PULP FRICTION

Remember that leftover celery pulp? Here's your chance to use it for a face and body scrub or leave it on longer for a restorative mask.

Ingredients

- 1 bunch celery (juiced) keep the pulp
- 1 cucumber
- 1 tbsp yoghurt
- 1 tbsp honey

Method

Juice the celery and cucumber. Remove the pulp by pouring the liquid through a strainer. Add the honey and yoghurt and mix well until it forms a paste. Apply to your face, neck, chest and arms in slow, circular motions. Leave on your skin for a longer treatment, removing with a face cloth and lukewarm water. Discard after use.

This is a great way to use up celery pulp from your morning's juice.
(Courtesy of Cottonbro/Pexels)

GO NUTS

The grainy texture of nuts and oats help to exfoliate your skin without irritation. This is ideal for sensitive skin, or if you have small areas of eczema or dermatitis (although test on an area first). The oil in the nuts helps to moisturise skin, while the oats remove the dead skin cells, revealing baby soft skin underneath. This is ideal for dry skin.

Ingredients

- 100mg ground nuts (try almonds or flax seeds)
- 50mg oatmeal
- 50mg whole wheat flour
- Water for paste (add gradually to get a consistency you prefer)

Method

Combine dry ingredients in a blender until they are reduced to a coarse mixture. Pour into an airtight glass jar. To use, scoop out a handful using a spoon, and place into a bowl, adding water to make a paste. Rub over your body to loosen any dry or flaking skin. By adding the water only when you use it, the mixture will keep for around six months.

LOVELY LADY HUMP-DAY SCRUB

If you have sensitive skin, or are prone to reactions, this grain-based scrub is ideal. Oatmeal is often used in baths or commercial scrubs for sensitive skin. Use just once a week.

Ingredients

- 2 tbsp oatmeal
- 2 tbsp cornmeal
- 2 tbsp wheatgerm

Method

Perfect for exfoliating normal to sensitive skin. Mix all ingredients together and store in an airtight container. Make a paste by adding a splash of warm water to one tablespoon of the mixture. Store in an airtight container but discard after one week.

BIG APPLE SCRUB

Apples contain antioxidants, which help the skin to renew itself. Using the fruit as part of an exfoliant allows new cells to emerge – your skin will look much fresher and smoother.
Ideal for normal or oily skin.

Ingredients

- 1 apple
- 2 tsp mineral water

Method

Juice the apple or blend until smooth. Add mineral water and pour into a bottle. Using a cotton wool ball, apply the lotion to your face, leaving for five to ten minutes. Rinse with lukewarm water and pat dry. Use within two weeks, storing in the refrigerator.

SKIN-SAVING SALVE

This is a great recipe to make up and keep for any cuts, bumps or bruises which need treating.

Ingredients
- 1 cup fresh or dried calendula flowers
- 1 cup olive oil
- 2 ounces beeswax
- ¼ tsp vitamin E (pierce two to three capsules for oil)
- 10 drops lemon essential oil

Method
Fill a jar with the flowers and pour in the oil until the flowers are completely covered. Allow the jar to sit in the sunlight for two to three weeks to allow the flowers to infuse the oil (shake every few days). After a few weeks, you can pour out the oil and store in an airtight container, discarding the flowers and any solid ingredients leftover.

CHAPTER NINE

YOUR DIY BEAUTY RECIPES FOR HAIR

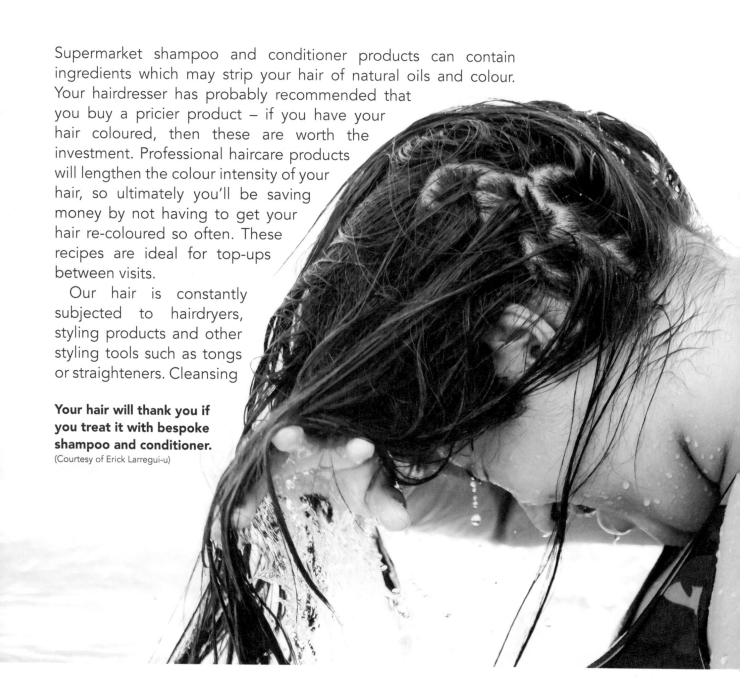

Supermarket shampoo and conditioner products can contain ingredients which may strip your hair of natural oils and colour. Your hairdresser has probably recommended that you buy a pricier product – if you have your hair coloured, then these are worth the investment. Professional haircare products will lengthen the colour intensity of your hair, so ultimately you'll be saving money by not having to get your hair re-coloured so often. These recipes are ideal for top-ups between visits.

Our hair is constantly subjected to hairdryers, styling products and other styling tools such as tongs or straighteners. Cleansing

Your hair will thank you if you treat it with bespoke shampoo and conditioner.
(Courtesy of Erick Larregui-u)

Parabens
Usually in skincare, some
haircare products contain
parabens, as they help
prevent bacteria forming in
the bottle.

Sulphates
Many shampoos use this
ingredient in order to create
bubbles or foam, yet they
can make your hair dry,
brittle and frizzy.

Fragrance
A shampoo which boasts
'essential oils' may cause
allergic reaction or
breathing issues. This is
because synthetic fragrances
can contain a number
of endocrine-disrupting
chemicals (EDCs), so
proceed with caution.

the hair and the scalp allows hair to 'breathe', rather like the skin on your face when it is cleansed. Removing excess oil from the scalp and the hair is necessary for healthy, shiny hair. It's up to you how often you wash your hair, as everyone is different.

SHAMPOO

NATURAL SHAMPOO BASE

This is a great base shampoo, to which you can add herbs or essential oils. Herbs can calm hair problems (such as frizzy hair or a tender scalp), while oils are vital to help coat the follicle to promote shine. Adding some herbs, such as chamomile, lavender or rose oil will also add a lovely scent to your hair. This shampoo can be used daily – or whenever you wash your hair.

Ingredients
¼ cup water
¼ cup castile soap [made from pure olive oil – most health food stores stock this]
½ tsp of (extra virgin) olive oil

Method
Mix together all ingredients and place into shampoo bottle. Shake well. Store in a tight container and discard after two weeks.

LAVENDER SHAMPOO

Lavender soothes an irritated scalp and stimulates the hair follicles. It also aids in relaxation and feelings of well-being. This is due to the scent released, which releases relaxing messages to the brain. Lavender is also extremely calming for the skin.

Ingredients
- ½ cup water
- ½ cup fresh lavender
- 2 tablespoons of glycerine
- ½ cup Natural Shampoo Base
- 5 drops of lavender essential oil

Method
Mix water and lavender together into a heavy bottom pot and bring to a boil. Boil gently for at least twenty minutes. Let the mixture

cool slightly and slowly add basic shampoo mixture and glycerine. Mix well. Pour shampoo into container and let the mixture stand until it thickens. Use as you would your regular shampoo. Can be kept for one month.

DANDRUFF ELIXIR

Tea tree is a must-have for everybody. It can be used to treat spots, cold sores and cuts, and is also ideal for treating nits. Tea tree eliminates snowy flakes by helping to remove build-up and chemical residues which can cause dandruff. It also controls the micro-organisms on our scalp, which may cause itchy flake syndrome. Best of all, it is ideal for those with sensitive scalps, so this mixture won't irritate your scalp as many commercial anti-dandruff brands can. You can use this mixture daily, or until your dandruff has disappeared.

Ingredients
- 4 or 5 drops tea tree oil
- 1 tbsp jojoba oil

Method
Combine the tea tree and jojoba oil into a glass jar and seal it with a lid. Shake the mixture well. After sectioning wet hair, dab mixture onto a clean cotton wad and stroke along the scalp. It's not necessary to use this product to the ends of the hair shaft, just the scalp where dandruff forms. Wrap hair in a towel and let sit for 2 hours. Work shampoo into hair with a little water to remove oil. Rinse. Discard mixture after one week.

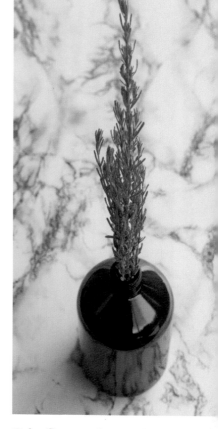

Calm flyaway hair and a busy mind with soothing lavender shampoo.
(Courtesy of Conleth Prosser)

CONDITIONER

The surface of your hair is made up of overlapping cuticles, like the tiles on a roof. These are 'lifted' by everyday activities like brushing and combing. Once lifted, they are vulnerable to damage, and expose the inside of your hair. Conditioner helps the cuticles lie flat and smoothing their edges to help prevent this kind of damage. As well as protecting your hair, this also makes it softer, more manageable and shinier. Using conditioner provides protection and helps to lock in moisture.

DRY HAIR CONDITIONER
Vinegar is an easy way to add shine to hair, as the acid in the vinegar

∽ TOP TIP ∽

If your hair is dry at the ends, but oily at the roots, only apply conditioner to the tips, so as not to overload the scalp with moisture.

helps to balance the oils of the follicle. Adding herbs, such as rosemary and mint are ideal for nourishing dry hair. Other nourishing oils are lemon, chamomile, peppermint or lime, all of which nourish the scalp, and provide calming and soothing properties.

This is a good recipe if you suffer from flyaway hair during the colder months as the vinegar helps to remove static.

Ingredients
- Handful of fresh rosemary
- Handful of fresh mint leaves
- 1 cup cider vinegar

Method
In a glass jar with a lid, place the rosemary and mint leaves and cover with the cider vinegar. Seal the jar and leave for two weeks. Strain the potion. After shampooing, pour a tablespoon onto dry hair and leave in. Use a wide-toothed combe to distribute the mixture evenly through to the ends of your hair. Use whenever you shampoo your hair. Discard after one month.

CONDITIONER FOR OILY HAIR
Like using lemon on your skin, lemon is an astringent that absorbs oil without damaging hair or follicles. Used repeatedly, this conditioner trains the hair follicles to release less oil, thus eliminating stringy, lifeless hair.

Ingredients
- 1 lemon
- ¼ cup apple cider vinegar

Method
Wash, slice, and de-seed the lemon. Squeeze the juice using a lemon squeezer or filter through a muslin to remove any pulp. Mix with the cider vinegar. After shampooing, blot hair with a towel and rub lemon-vinegar mixture into scalp. Leave on for around five to ten minutes then rinse with cool water. Use after shampooing. If your hair is excessively oily, use every other day. Discard any excess mixture.

IN IT FOR THE LONG HAUL
Increase the shine of your hair with these essential oils. I'd recommend using this at night for extra conditioning time, for

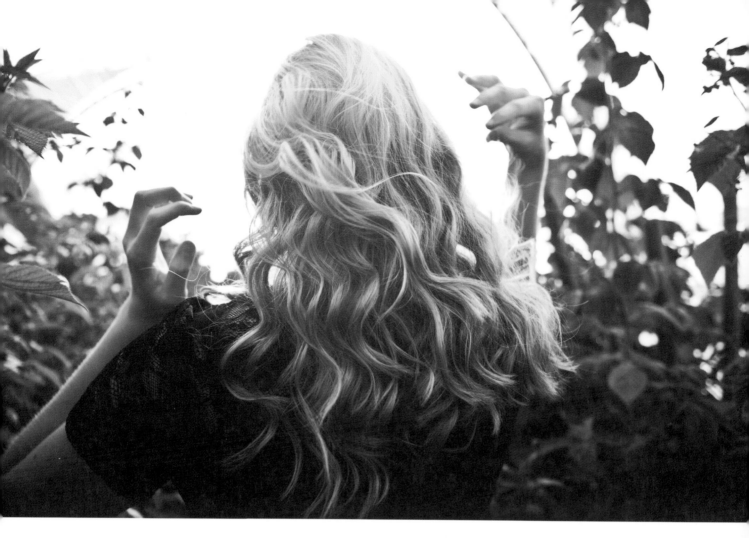

extra treatments, plus the essential oils are known for their relaxing properties, so you'll sleep well. The oils work by coating the hair shaft, encouraging the follicles to lie flat. When these are flat, light is reflected off the hair, creating an illusion of shiny hair. By leaving the oils on your hair overnight, they will have the opportunity to penetrate deeper. Some oils, such as rosemary are invigorating and stimulating, which may promote hair growth. If your hair is dry or lifeless, use this treatment once a week and always keep it on overnight.

Essential oils can add some much-needed shine to dry hair.
(Courtesy of Tim Mossholder)

Ingredients
- 3 drops neroli oil
- 3 drops chamomile essential oil
- 3 drops lavender essential oil
- 3 drops rosemary essential oil

Method
Mix the ingredients in a small bowl. Shampoo hair as normal. Towel dry and apply the mixture. Comb through and allow to dry naturally. For deeper treatment, wear a shower cap or apply cling film around

your head. Don't forget to place a towel on your pillow! Discard any excess mixture.

HAIR COLOURANT

While you can't bleach your hair using natural ingredients, nor permanently dye it, there are ways to subtly change the tone or highlight your hair.

BLONDE MOMENTS HIGHLIGHTER

This will give you a very subtle highlight, particularly if your hair is naturally light anyway.

Ingredients
- 10 chamomile teabags
- Juice of 1 lemon
- 800ml boiling water

Method

Steep the teabags in boiling water. Remove the bags and add the lemon juice. Cool. After shampooing your hair pour the concoction over your hair and work it through your hair to the ends. Leave throughout the day (braid your hair to keep it tidy) and shampoo out the next time you shower. You can keep any leftover for up to one week in an airtight bottle or container.

DARK PHASE TINT TREATMENT

A full hair dye or change of colour is best left to the professionals, or permanent products, but this recipe will give your locks a glossy sheen, helping it appear fuller, thicker and shinier.

Ingredients
- ½ cup dried sage
- 250ml boiling water

Method

Steep the sage in the boiling water for around 30 minutes – 1 hour. Cool, then pour the liquid through a strainer. Pour the sage water over your freshly washed hair and leave for 15 to 30 minutes. Rinse out and apply conditioner for extra shine. Discard any mixture you didn't use.

SIGN OF THE TIMES

If you want to cover up your grey hair in between salon treatments, you can use this great coffee mix, to temporarily mask them.

Ingredients

- ½ cup of coffee
- 2 tbsp coffee grounds
- 1 cup coconut oil

Method

Mix ingredients together and pour into a jar. Shake well. Apply to your hair after shampooing and leave in for at least sixty minutes. Rinse out (don't use shampoo) and style as usual. Discard any excess.

HAIR MASKS

Taking time to treat your hair is just as important as pampering your skin. Most of these hair masks require around one hour to seep into the hair follicle. For extra conditioning, wrap your hair in cling film, or a hot towel (heat it in the microwave). Use this time to read, relax or meditate, or apply a face mask for a double treat.

BANANA HAIR MASK

Bananas help restore shine and vitality to your hair, and the olive oil will help smooth cuticles.

Ingredients

1 ripe banana
1 tbsp olive oil

Method

Mash the bananas in a bowl with a fork and add oil. Apply the mixture to wet hair, from the roots to the ends. Massage all the way through your hair – it's a good time to give yourself a head massage at the same time. This will also help stimulate hair growth. Wrap your hair in cling film, or a hot towel (heat it in the microwave). Rinse with warm water before shampooing and conditioning. If you have any leftover throw it away as it won't keep.

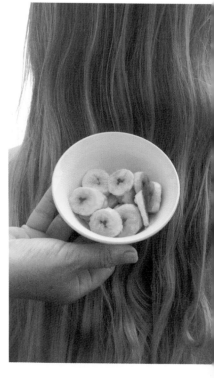

If your hair has had too much fun in the sun this will help restore smooth locks.
(Courtesy of Conleth Prosser)

HOT HAIR MASK

For exceptionally dry hair, this hair mask treatment will help restore softness. If your hair is dry with split ends, visit a hairdresser for a trim. You'll notice the difference immediately.

Ingredients
• 3 tablespoons pure jojoba oil

Method
Place the jojoba oil into a pitcher, such as a milk jug. Warm the oil in the microwave and apply it to your hair (check first that it's not too hot), starting at the ends and working up to the top of head. Wrap hair in a towel and relax for an hour or leave the oil in overnight. Rinse and shampoo hair as usual. This is a great once-a-week treatment.

AVOCADO HAIR MASK

With its natural oils, the avocado is one of the miracle workers of Mother Nature's cupboard. This hair mask is ideal for dry or normal hair.

Ingredients
1 avocado
1 tbsp olive oil (if desired)

Method
Mash the avocado in a bowl, adding the oil to the mixture. Apply to your hair, beginning at the roots, working it all the way through to the ends. Cover with a shower cap, and a hot towel if desired and relax for 30 minutes. Rinse with warm water. Shampoo and condition as normal. Avocados won't keep so you'll need to discard any excess.

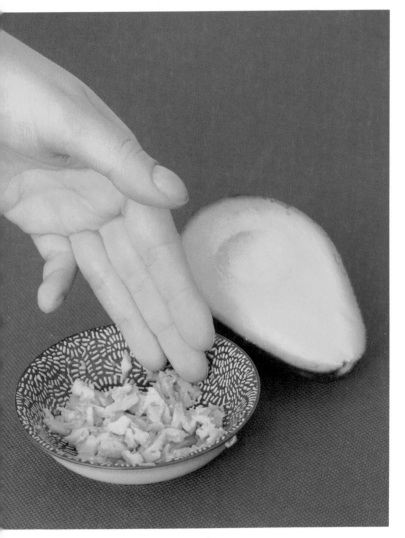

Dry, frizzy hair needs some extra moisture. Avocado is the perfect ingredient to restore some shine. (Courtesy of Conleth Prosser)

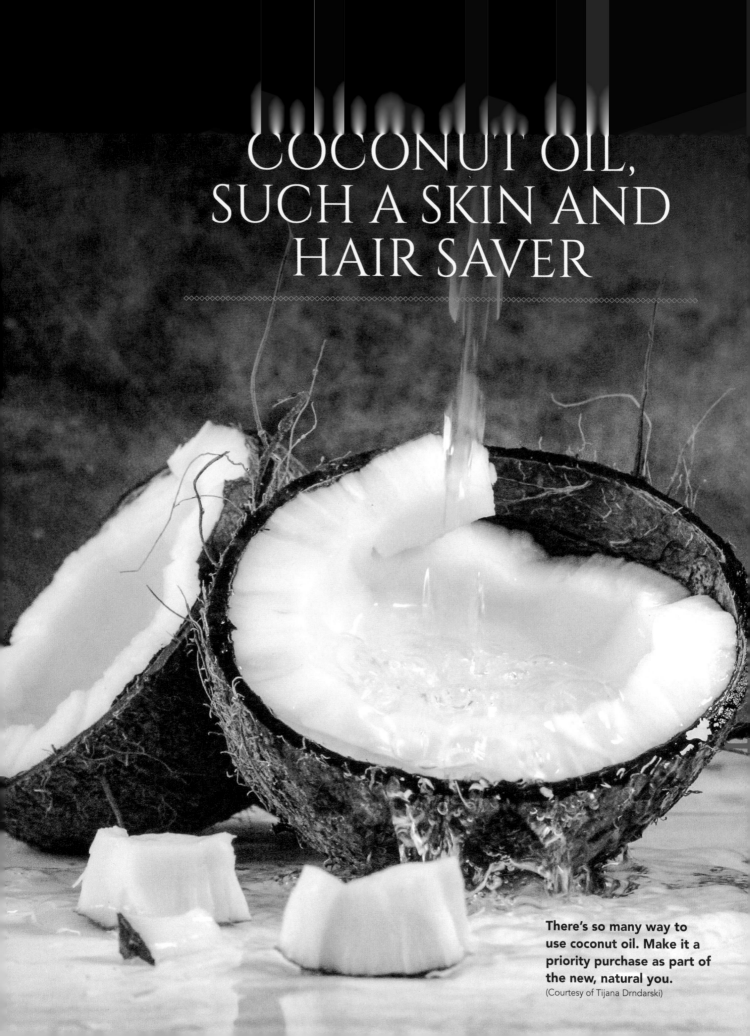

COCONUT OIL, SUCH A SKIN AND HAIR SAVER

There's so many way to use coconut oil. Make it a priority purchase as part of the new, natural you.
(Courtesy of Tijana Drndarski)

Why coconut oil is a god

You can use coconut oil for so many beauty treatments. Try these for top-to-toe treatments:

COCONUT FOR YOUR NOGGIN

Coconut oil is ideal for a hair treatment as it easily penetrates the hair shaft, giving it smoothness and shine. Apply a small amount to your palm, then to the ends of your hair, working the produce back towards your scalp. Comb through and pop on a shower cap while you relax over a book. Leave overnight for particularly dry hair. You will probably need

Coconut oil penetrates the hair shaft to help restore your strands to their shining glory.

(Courtesy of Biome.com.au)

DID YOU KNOW?

If your hair tends towards frizz, apply a tiny amount of coconut to the ends. Rub between your fingers to warm it up then apply to the perm-tastic tangles.

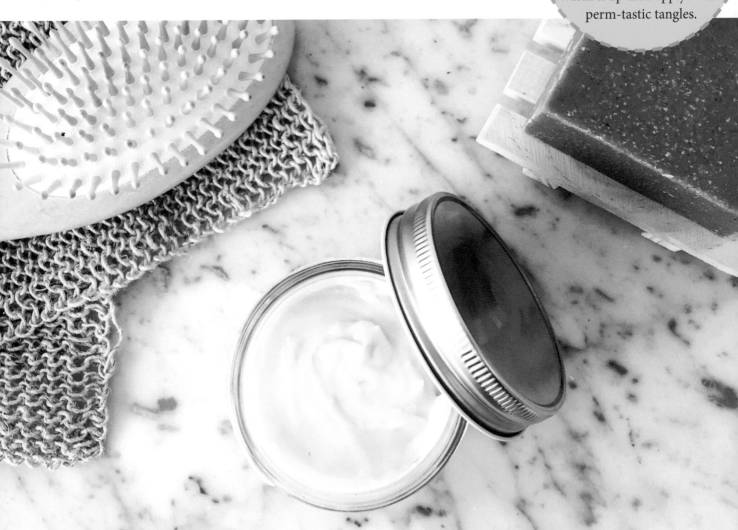

to shampoo your hair twice the next morning to remove the oil completely. This will leave your hair shiny, but not oily.

COCONUT FOR YOUR FACE

Face wash
Rub some coconut oil into your cleansed skin, pressing firmly in circular motions, beginning at the jaw line and moving towards the hairline. Cleanse with warm water and a face cloth.

FACE FACTS COCONUT MASK

Ingredients
- 2 tbsp melted coconut oil
- Juice of a lemon
- Honey (organic, local or manuka is best)

Method
Mix the ingredients in a bowl and apply to clean skin. Leave for around 15 minutes, before removing with lukewarm water, wipes or a soft cloth.

LOVELY LIPS SCRUB
Remove dead skin from your lips with this nourishing lip scrub. Peppermint oil adds a tasty zing but use whichever essential oil you prefer.

TOP TIP

For some lovely scented locks, add rosemary, lavender or sandalwood essential oil to the coconut.

DID YOU KNOW?

Coconut oil is a great and gentle way to remove eye makeup, especially if you've worn mascara. It'll whisk your eye products away without irritation.

Soften dry, flaky lips with this lip balm. The mint will add an extra tingle.
(Courtesy of Conleth Prosser)

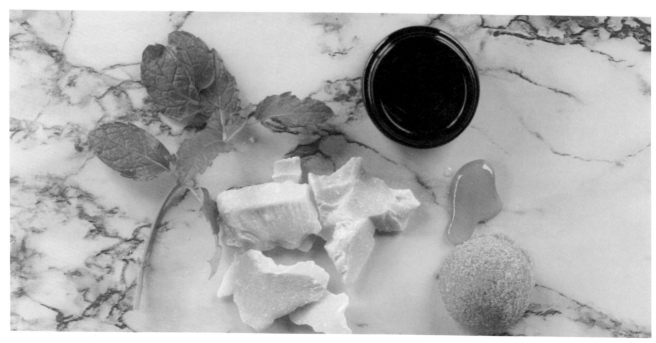

Ingredients

- 1 tbsp coconut oil
- 1 tsp brown sugar
- 1 tsp honey
- 1 drop peppermint oil

Method

Mix products together in a small jar with a sealable lid. Apply to your lips, gently rubbing to remove any dead skin cells or flakes. Rinse off. Add a dab of coconut oil for some extra moisture.

LOVELY LIP BALM

Boast kissable lips with this wonderfully nourishing lip treatment.

Ingredients

- 2 tbsp coconut oil
- 2 tbsp cocoa butter
- 2 tbsp grated beeswax or beeswax pellets
- Cinnamon, lavender or peppermint essential oil

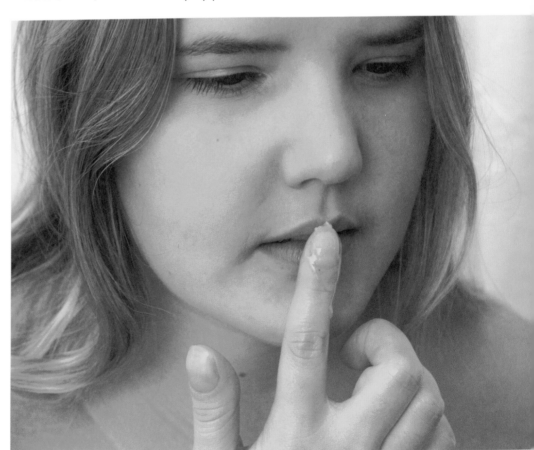

Apply lip balm as often as you need it. These natural ingredients won't dry out your lips.
(Courtesy of Conleth Prosser)

Method

Combine the coconut oil, cocoa butter and beeswax into a heat resistant measuring jug. Pour 25ml water into the cup and heat in the microwave, for one minute at a time, stirring each time until all the ingredients are combined. Remove from the microwave and pour the mixture into a small glass proof lip container or jar. Add two drops of your chosen essential oil and stir with a teaspoon or chopstick. Seal and refrigerate immediately.

COCONUTTY BODY SCRUB

You'll emerge from the shower with gorgeously soft, silky skin. Add an essential oil such as eucalyptus, peppermint or sandalwood for a delicious treat.

Ingredients

- ½ cup coconut oil
- 1 cup brown sugar
- Five drops of your chosen essential oil

Or

- 2 drops vanilla extract

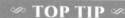

∽ TOP TIP ∽

Coconut oil can be used on its own for dry hands and cuticles.

Method

Combine all the ingredients into a saucepan, and melt the coconut oil on a low heat, stirring continuously. Add the essential oil or essence, allow to cool then apply when you're in the shower. Rinse well and either use coconut oil as a moisturiser afterwards or jojoba oil to seal in the hydration.

A TREAT FOR YOUR FEET

If the soles of your feet are cracked, sore, or you've been suffering from a fungal infection, coconut oil is a wonderful way to restore softness and banish any lingering bacteria. Apply coconut oil directly to your feet and pop some cotton socks on. Wear overnight. Repeat this treatment around three times a week.

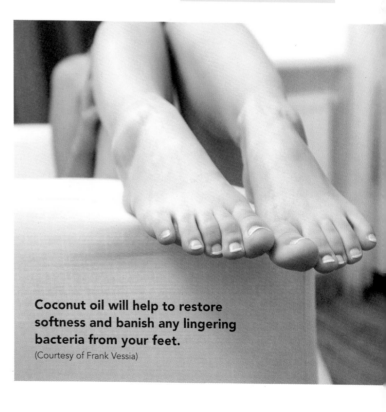

Coconut oil will help to restore softness and banish any lingering bacteria from your feet.
(Courtesy of Frank Vessia)

CHAPTER ELEVEN

FACIALS AND MASSAGES

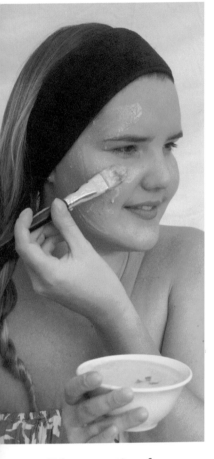

Take some time for yourself and enjoy a facial, hair mask and body treatment.
(Courtesy of Conleth Prosser)

TAKING REGULAR TIME to enjoy facials and moisturisers can go a long way to help you reduce stress, treat skin or hair irritations and deal with any beauty problems. While nothing can beat a facial or a massage performed by a professional, you can still pamper yourself by learning the right way to cleanse, exfoliate and treat your skin. Massages, especially foot, hand or head massages, can also be done by yourself.

Before you start
Blend the carrier and essential oil well by shaking the jar vigorously. Don't apply directly to the skin (it'll drip onto the floor and make a mess): instead, pour a small amount into your hand and rub your palms together. This warms up the oil and blends the ingredients further.

HOW TO

HEAD MASSAGES
You know that 'aaah' feeling you get when you're at the hairdressers and they take some time to massage your scalp between the shampoo and conditioning stage? A scalp massage helps to stimulate growth and can relief any stress or tension store in your temples or neckline.

Step 1. You can use oil or dry hands for this scalp massage. Either warm up the oil in your palm or rub your hands together to create heat.

Step 2. Place your face in your hands, breathing deeply. Then slowly run your fingers over your face, into your scalp.

Step 3. Move your fingers firmly in large, rotating circles, pressing firmly against the scalp.

Step 4. Continue from your forehead towards the back of your head. Rest your head against your thumb – this will help reduce the tension at the base of your neck.

Step 5. Repeat as often as you like.

FACE MASSAGE

Sometimes our skin can appear tired, puffy, bloated or dry. A quick facial massage is a good way to increase circulation – you can use your serum for this.

Step 1. Heat the oil between your palms by rubbing them together.

Step 2. Beginning at your chest, slowly rub the oil in, using sweeping circular movements to massage the oil in. Then, using upward movements, massage the oil into the neck, then along the jaw area, focusing on one side, then the other. Finish off with your fingers firmly pressing the oil into your forehead, gently massaging as though pulling bread apart.

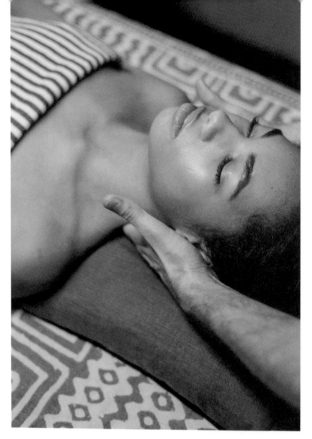

Restore glow and vitality with a facial, designed to help improve circulation and even tone.
(Courtesy of Cottonbro/Pexels)

MASSAGE OILS AND ADDITIONS

Massage and treatments are where essential oils really come into their own. You can choose your own base, or carrier oil, and add a few drops of your favourite oil for the outcome you like. A word of warning, never apply essential oils directly to the skin, as it can cause irritations or even burn your skin. Dilute it well in your carrier oil.

Remember: essential oils are highly concentrated extracts. Make sure that you always dilute them before applying to skin. If you do get any essential oil in your eyes, rinse them with a few drops of pure sweet almond oil. Water doesn't mix with oil.

Never drink or digest essential oils without first diluting them. Always check before using in cooking or in drinks.

Keep to the recommended dose. Some essential oils are toxic in large amounts so you should never increase the dose.

Some essential oils should not be used by pregnant women, or on children under the age of 2. The general advice is to avoid all essential oils during the first two trimesters.

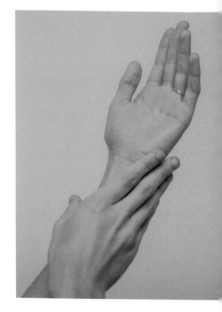

Even a short hand massage can help improve circulation and even help banish headaches.
(Courtesy of Juan Pablo Serrano Arenas)

Enjoy:
Lavender
Chamomile
Ylang Ylang
Eucalyptus
Geranium
Ginger
Grapefruit
Juniper
Lemon
Mandarin
Neroli
Rose
Sandalwood
Orange
Tea tree

Avoid:
Cinnamon
Clove
Rosemary
Clary sage
Jasmine

*NOTE: Do not go out in the sun for at least 6 hours after using any of the following oils in your recipes: ginger, lemon, orange and bergamot, as they can cause skin irritations if exposed to sun. Ideally, use these oils at night.

SOME WORDS ON OILS

Carrier oils
Carrier oils are vegetable oils used to dilute the concentrated essential oils and they help to slow down the evaporation of the

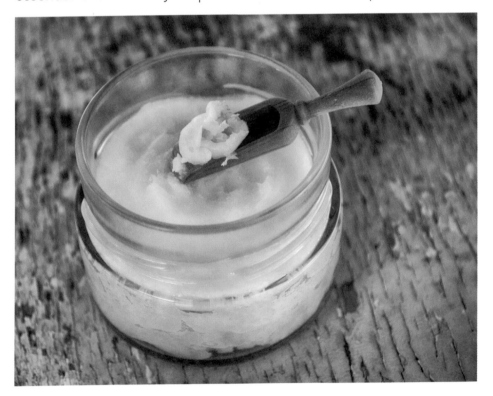

Oils are what your skin, hair and body needs to look its best.
(Courtesy of Biome.com.au)

essential oils and help absorb them into the skin. They should be extra virgin or cold-pressed vegetable oils for maximum benefit.

Some good carrier oils include mineral oil, grapeseed, safflower, sunflower, sesame, wheatgerm, olive or peanut oil.

Vegetable oil
A great base oil, best used to condition hair and nails.

Shea butter
I'm a big fan of shea butter, so if you're buying it, do so in bulk. As you can use it on its own without even adding anything further, it's a good bathroom beauty basic. Remember it's deeply moisturising, so best for areas such as feet, elbows or extremely dry skin

Massage oils
Using an oil when massaging is not just for comfort and for hydrating the skin, oils contain many healing properties, including relaxation, detoxification, skin-repair and revitalisation. It is recommended that you familiarise yourself with the properties of any oil you are intending to use, as well as discover whether a particular oil works best when combined with another.

Essential oils, when added to a carrier (massage) oil, are excellent healers and can be used in many ways. They can be used for face and body massage, added to a warm bath or burnt in an oil dish to release their aroma. Some oils can even be used neat to help heal burns and scars.

Storing
Store essential oils in brown or dark blue glass bottles with a close fitting plastic screw cap. Do not store in plastic containers, they could become contaminated. Keep them in a dark, cool place to prolong the shelf life. Always store out of reach of children.

BASIC MASSAGE OIL RECIPE

If you've never made your own massage oil, this is a good place to start. As you become familiar with the various oils and their properties you can become more adventurous with your mixtures. A good oil to begin with is lavender oil: it is an excellent addition to a base oil and can be added to a bath to aid relaxation or used before bed for those who suffer from insomnia or sleeping difficulties.

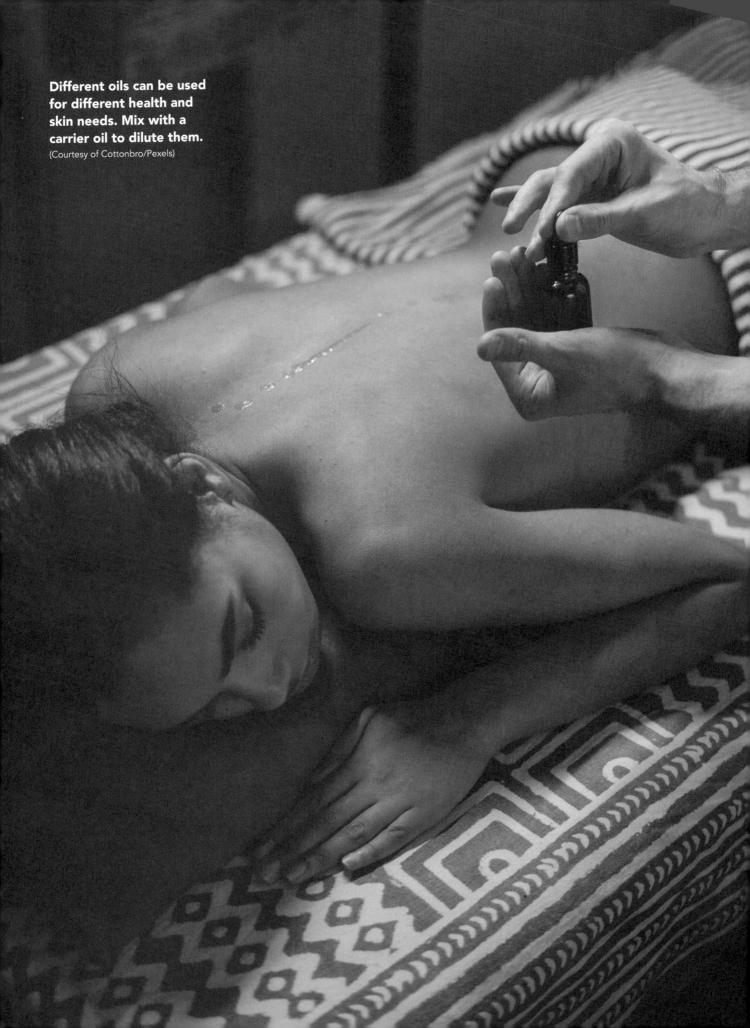

Different oils can be used for different health and skin needs. Mix with a carrier oil to dilute them.
(Courtesy of Cottonbro/Pexels)

Ingredients
- 6 tsp carrier oil of your choice
- 8 drops of oil of your choice

Method
Blend ingredients well in a clean bottle. Replace the cap and shake well. Warm up oil before doing any massage including your fingertips.

SUGGESTED RECIPES FOR SPECIAL MASSAGE OILS

REFRESHING MASSAGE OIL
Rose and jasmine are uplifting oils. Use this blend if you are suffering from headaches or are feeling down.

Ingredients
- 6–8 tsp grapeseed oil
- 6 drops of lavender oil
- 2 drops rose oil
- 2 drops jasmine oil

Method
Blend essential oils with the grapeseed oil. Use this oil on your temples or give yourself a relaxing foot massage before bedtime.

SLEEPY HEAD MASSAGE OIL
If you're having trouble falling asleep or staying asleep at night, this blend will encourage relaxation. Chamomile and lavender are popular oils to encourage sleepiness and rose and jasmine help to reduce feelings of stress and anxiety.

Ingredients
- 10 tsp grapeseed oil
- 6 drops of chamomile oil
- 4 drops jasmine oil
- 2 drops rose oil
- 1 drop lavender oil

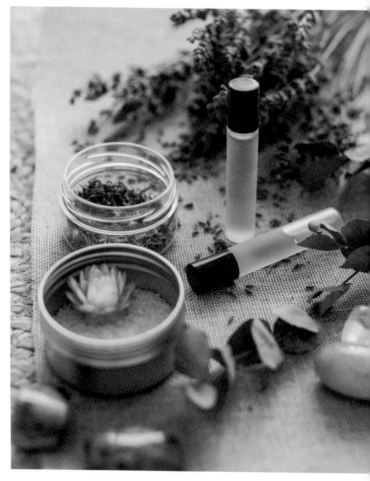

Use lavender essential oil in your bath, sprinkled on your pillow or dab some on your temples for a good night's sleep. (Courtesy of Katya Alagich)

Method

Add the oils to the grapeseed oil. If you suffer from severe sleeplessness, drop a few drops of lavender oil onto your pillow before going to bed.

IN THE MOOD MASSAGE OIL

This uplifting, yet relaxing oil is a good combination if you're planning a lazy romantic evening with your partner. Give your partner a massage to get them in the mood (but make sure it's reciprocated).

Ingredients
- 10 tsp oil (of your choice)
- 5 drops of lavender oil
- 2 drops chamomile oil
- 2 drops frankincense oil
OR
- 2 drops rose oil
- 2 drops jasmine oil

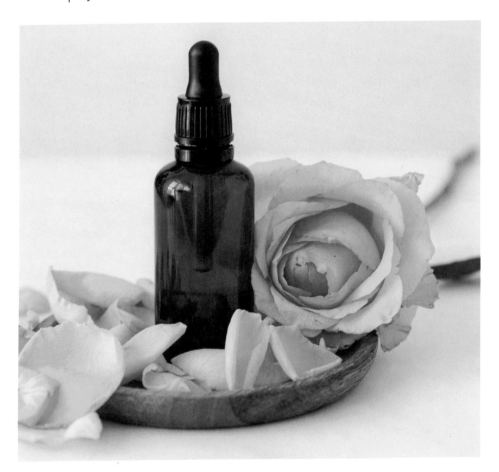

Learn how to give your partner a massage. The pay off? They have to return the favour.
(Courtesy of Karolina Grabowska)

Method

Add the essential oils to the oil and blend well. Use this oil for a relaxing neck, shoulder and back massage.

SOMETHING SPICY MASSAGE OIL

If you're feeling a little under the weather, this is the ideal oil for you. Myrrh and eucalyptus are an excellent essential oils if you have a cold or blocked sinus.

Ingredients
- 6–8 tsp grapeseed oil
- 6 drops of sandalwood oil
- 2 drops myrrh oil
- 2 drops eucalyptus
- 2 drops jasmine oil

Method

This essential oil blend can be used in the bath, or as a steam to help clear your head. Add a few drops to boiling water and inhale for five minutes.

STRESS RELIEF MASSAGE OIL

If you, like the majority of society, are suffering from signs of stress, then try using this oil blend in your bath or as a massage oil on your hands or feet before going to bed. Petitgrain helps lift the spirits and relieve anxiety.

Ingredients
- 8 tsp grapeseed oil
- 3 drops lavender
- 2 drops petitgrain
- 1–2 drops frankincense

Method

Add the oils to the grapeseed oil and blend well. If you're having a particularly difficult or stressful time, or having trouble sleeping, add five drops to an aromatherapy burner at work or in your bedroom.

R-E-L-A-X MASSAGE OIL

Lavender is the staple essential oil, which everyone should have in their bathroom cabinet, as it helps relieve most signs of stress and insomnia.

Ingredients
- 8 tsp safflower oil
- 4 drops lavender
- 1 drop petitgrain
- 1 drop frankincense

Method
Add essential oils to the safflower oil and massage temples, neck and balls of your feet. Then it's time to say 'sleep-tight'!

JOINT RELIEF MASSAGE OIL

Ginger is one of the best oils you can use if you're affected by arthritis, as it is extremely therapeutic. The combination of juniper and rosemary – also helpful for arthritis – is ideal, particularly if you're dealing with backache.

Ingredients
- 8 tsp sunflower oil
- 3 drops white birch
- 3 drops ginger
- 2 drops juniper
- 3 drops rosemary

Method
This blend can be added to cream or oil and applied to sore and inflamed joints.

OUT OF THE COLD MASSAGE OIL

Eucalyptus is one of the best ways I've found to stop a cold in its tracks. Marjoram will also help to relieve the aches and pains associated with colds and flu.

Ingredients
- 8 tbsp wheatgerm oil
- 2 drops eucalyptus
- 2 drops lavender
- 2 drops marjoram

Method
If you're giving someone a massage and they have a cold, make sure their body is nice and warm, even the parts you aren't massaging. Heat towels in the microwave to cover body parts which aren't being treated or use hot water bottles.

Or use the essential oils listed for a steam or in the bath to help your recovery.

BE HAPPY MASSAGE OIL

This uplifting blend is helped by the addition of the stress-relieving ylang ylang oil. Sandalwood is also a good anxiety-reliever, plus it's excellent for cellulite and improving circulation in the legs.

Ingredients

- 12 tsp safflower oil
- 2 drops bergamot
- 2 drops geranium
- 3 drops jasmine
- 2 drops petitgrain
- 2 drops rose
- 2 drops sandalwood
- 3 drops ylang ylang

Method

Add the essential oils to the carrier oil and store in a glass container in a cool, dry place. You can use the oil in the shower to massage in with a body brush or loofah or apply after bathing as part of your moisturising treatments. Add a couple of drops to your body cream to carry the happy vibe with you all day long.

PEACE OF MIND MASSAGE OIL

Neroli and Melissa oils are extremely relaxing oils, and their effect is almost immediate. Neroli is also an excellent oil to apply to your temples or bath if you're suffering from a hangover.

Ingredients

- 12 tsp wheatgerm carrier oil
- 2 drops geranium
- 3 drops lavender
- 2 drops marjoram
- 3 drops Melissa
- 2 drops neroli
- 2 drops tangerine
- 3 drops ylang ylang.

Method

Try using this oil on your temples before a busy workday or after a stressful day. Burn it at home to help create a calm environment for your family, or in your bath before bedtime.

SERENITY MASSAGE OIL

Ingredients
- 8 tbsp carrier oil
- 3 drops clary sage
- 3 drops lavender
- 2 drops marjoram
- 2 drops petitgrain
- 3 drops ylang ylang

Method
Mix the ingredients together and apply to the stress points – the neck, back of the knees, shoulders or add to a bath or oil burner for some olfactory release.

TAKE A DEEP BREATH MASSAGE OIL
Do not use before bed as this oil is mildly stimulating, but it's an ideal one to use in the morning to get your day off to a great start.

Ingredients
- 2 tbsp carrier oil
- 2 drops eucalyptus
- 2 drops lavender
- 2 drops peppermint

Method
Combine the ingredients and mix well. You can use this as a body oil, inhalation (add some drops to extremely hot water for a quick morning steam, or in a warm bath.

A head massage can help relieve tension headaches.
(Courtesy of Andrea Piacquadio)

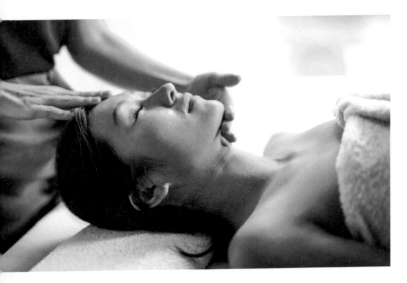

REVIVING HEAD MASSAGE
Particularly good for relieving headaches, especially those caused by stress, tension or muscle pain in the neck and shoulders.

Ingredients
2 tbsp carrier oil
2 drops lavender oil
2 drops peppermint oil

Method
Apply to the temples or base of skull for relief.

HOW TO DO A DIY FACIAL

A face massage should be done daily to help ward off the signs of ageing. Many people swear by daily or regular facial exercises. But by applying your moisturiser or facial oil with a massage technique you'll help the product sink into your skin and give yourself a relaxing treat at the same time.

Step 1. Apply a hair band or shower cap to keep your hair off your face

Step 2. Warm up the facial oil or cleanser in your hand. This will activate the ingredients and help them sink into your skin.

Step 3. Beginning at your neck, gently massage from your neck, up towards your chin.

Step 4. Bring your thumb and forefinger together in a slightly 'pinching' movement, lifting the skin up very gently and lightly along your jaw line towards your earlobe, continuing to press the oil into your skin.

Step 5. Repeat on the other side.

Step 6. Begin moving upwards. From the outer corner of your lip repeat the above pinching and pressing movement towards your ear.

Step 7. Repeat on the other side.

Step 8. Massage from the base of your nostril towards the temple, up over your cheekbone.

Step 9. Repeat on the other side

Step 10. Press firmly on the fleshy part on other side of the nose, to help reduce puffiness and congestion in the sinus area.

Step 11. Massage the forehead, continuing the strokes upwards towards your hairline.

Step 12. Massage your ears, beginning at the tips and ending at the earlobes with a slight squeeze.

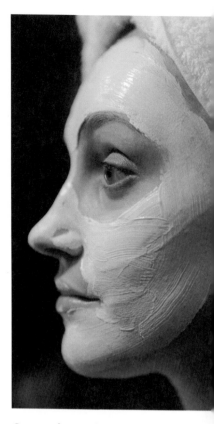

Correctly applying cleansers, moisturisers and face masks can help increase their potency.
(Courtesy of Cottonbro/Pexels)

CHAPTER TWELVE

TIPS, TRICKS, SOS AND DOS AND DON'TS OF DIY BEAUTY

QUICK DIY SOS TREATMENTS AND TRICKS

Free cold coffee

If you've made yourself a large jug of coffee and have some left over, don't waste it. Instead, pour it into your ice cube tray and freeze. Use when your eye area needs some TLC after a late night. The caffeine (and cold!) helps to stimulate circulation around the eye area.

Go green

Green tea bags contain antioxidants – they're a healthy alternative to your regular tea or coffee, and may help control weight, increase energy and keep the signs of ageing at bay. Soak the tea bags in cool water and apply to your eyes. Lie down for five ten minutes while they work their magic. Remove and rinse your face with cold water.

Vitamin E capsules

This is mentioned in the recipes, but vitamin E capsules are a facelift in the bottle. Vitamin E supplements contain pure oil, which is extremely hydrating and has antioxidant and anti-ageing properties. Pierce a vitamin E capsule at night and apply to clean skin.

Plant some aloe vera

This wonder plant is great for treating burns, cold sores, sunburn, and heated, good for sore joints. You can grow aloe vera from a cutting of another plant. Water sparingly and just snap off a small piece. The thick juice – with a similar consistency to honey – will ooze. Use this on the affected area.

Fast and fabulous face mask

If you've only got ten minutes to spare but your skin is crying out for some love, whip up this instance facial treatment. Mix two parts yoghurt with one part honey. Apply to your face and leave for ten minutes. Rinse and apply serum and moisturiser to your glowing skin.

THINGS TO AVOID IN DIY BEAUTY

The beauty gurus at the Australian Skin Clinic kindly shared their top tips on what you can and shouldn't do to your skin at home.

1. DIY Don't: use charcoal in a mask or commercial charcoal peel-off masks

Charcoal is a known detoxifying ingredient with cleansing properties, but the physical action of removing these peel-off masks can contribute to the tearing of collagen, elastin and other fibres, causing micro-trauma to the skin. The charcoal also loses its detoxifying and cleansing properties when combined with glue, meaning the masks can draw out oil and moisture from the skin, potentially leading to a drier complexion.

The alternative: a much more effective way of reducing pore size and clearing up blackheads is by using products with AHA natural ingredients.

2. DIY Don't: using hairspray to 'set' your makeup

Hairspray is fantastic for setting the perfect curl, or keeping wispy hair off your neck or ears, but should it be used to set makeup? NO WAY! Not only does hairspray contain alcohol and other unhealthy ingredients, it can cause skin to become dehydrated and dry. This often results in an irritated, itchy and red complexion as well as leaving your make up with a sticky feeling. Regular use could also lead to breakouts.

The alternative: Makeup setting sprays should sit weightlessly on the skin to prevent smudging and control oils, deflect surface shine and keep the skin looking matte. If your skin is looking a little oily you can use those disposable toilet seat covers to mop up any slick.

3. DIY Don't: Using milk of magnesia as a primer

Milk of magnesia is often used for stomach health and as a deodorant,

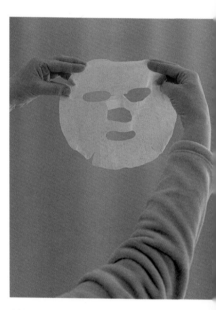

Sheet masks are a great way to infuse extra moisture into your skin.
(Courtesy of Anna Shvets)

but it has started trending as a makeup primer for oily skin. No matter what skin type you have, using Milk of magnesia on your face is a no-no in our books! Naturally, our skin is slightly acidic and we have an acidic mantle that stops bad bacteria penetrating the skin. Milk of magnesia has a high pH that can damage this acidic mantle, allowing nasty bacteria to get past the skin's defences and cause acne and dry skin. With the skin unable to shed its dead layers, clogged pores and breakouts can occur and cause further damage to skin's overall integrity.

The alternative: The goal of a primer is to optimise the skin's surface before makeup application, allowing makeup to look smoother and last longer. Well-hydrated skin is less likely to draw moisture from liquid foundation, so if you don't have any primer on hand, a normal moisturiser or even a spot control serum can work as a substitute.

4. DIY Don't: DIY Sugar Waxing

Sugar waxing is the 'old-is-new' way to remove hair with things you already have around the house. It is made from food substances like toffee and aims to remove hair by the root. While this may sound tempting, especially when stuck at home and unable to come in for your laser hair removal appointment, sugar waxing is only effective for specific hair lengths and can cause skin inflammation, bacterial infections and burns on the skin if performed incorrectly.

The alternative: Shave your legs is the best option to stay smooth, without disrupting your hair-growth cycle.

A FEW HOME BEAUTY QUESTIONS ANSWERED

Are derma rollers worth it?

If you're a fan of Instagram and follow any beauty gurus, you'll may have seen them brandishing what looks like a tiny lawnmower, complete with equally small needles. This is called a derma-rolling and promises to deliver brand new, youthful skin. It involves rolling micro-needles along your skin – the needles make microscopic incisions in the skin, creating a 'trauma'. The skin then goes into 'repair mode' by stimulating collagen production.

Use a Derma-roller three times a week at night after applying your toner and then once you've tested the product a few times and your skin's reaction to it, you can increase the frequency to nightly.

Are Gua sha tools worth investing in?

You may also have seen these flat jade or rose crystal 'smoothers' for sale or on your social media feed. Gua sha are angled stones – usually

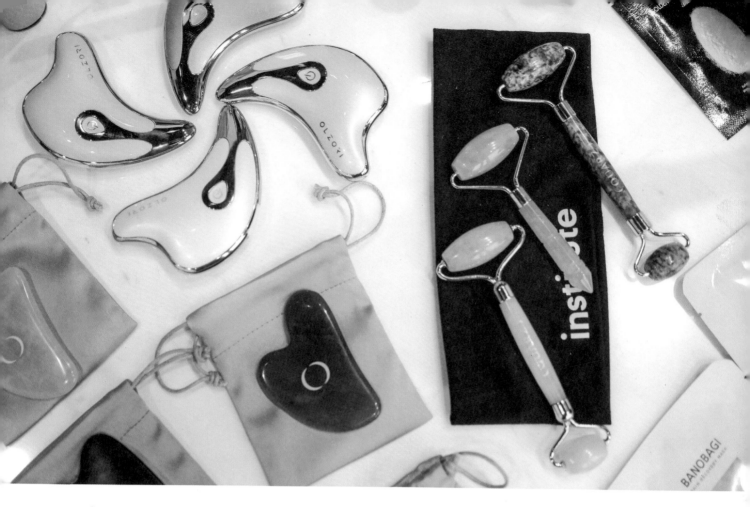

made out of crystal, bone or horn – the tool is used to firmly scrape the skin on the face to promote blood flow and energy redirection. Boasting claims of bright, improved skin, as well as a 'natural facelift,' they're the new anti-ageing tool kept by those who are serious about their skincare.

But do they work?

Gua sha is an ancient Chinese practice for energy flow and blood circulation. Typically they were used over the entire body, until the skin was reddened, but the new technique is to use the tool for soothing and massaging.

The benefits are numerous. Enthusiasts of Gua sha tools say that they notice an improvement in blood circulation (some studies suggest an increase of up to 400 per cent), lymphatic draining and skin elasticity and a reduction in the appearance of wrinkles.

If nothing else, the mere massaging technique you use to help your skin better absorb the serum is a relaxing regime to follow.

Gua sha tools or jade rollers may all help the product sink into your skin more effectively.

(Courtesy of Polina Tankilevitch/Pexels)

How to use

Hold the gua sha at a 45 degree angle. Softly 'dragging' the tool, as though scraping the skin, follow an upwards and outwards motion, starting at the centre of the face, and working your way outwards. Use the pointy part of the stone to gently massage deeper wrinkles. Continue the massage for one to three minutes morning and night.

CHAPTER THIRTEEN

DIY MAKEUP

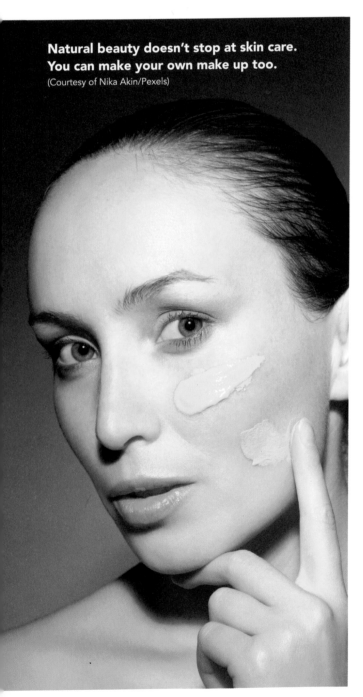

Natural beauty doesn't stop at skin care. You can make your own make up too.
(Courtesy of Nika Akin/Pexels)

IF YOU'RE TRULY serious about following a naturally beautiful lifestyle, then this may extend to using make up you've created yourself. A benefit of making your own means that you can create your own shades. If you experience allergies and reactions to mass-produced beauty products, this may be an answer to your problems.

Some make up ingredients, such as talc, zinc and bismuth, may cause skin irritations and eczema, particularly around the eyes. As with any beauty product, homemade or shop bought, they should be discarded after three months.

EYE SHADOW

If you tend to react to eyeshadow, this may be a way to add depth or colour to your makeup.

Ingredients
• Arrowroot powder

Then add whichever colour you desire for your eye shadow. Use as much or as little as you like according to the shade you're after. If you prefer your eye shadow to be cream-based, you can use 1/8 tsp of shea butter to the arrowroot powder.

• Brown– cocoa powder
• Green – spirulina
• Black/grey – activated charcoal
• Golden brown – nutmeg

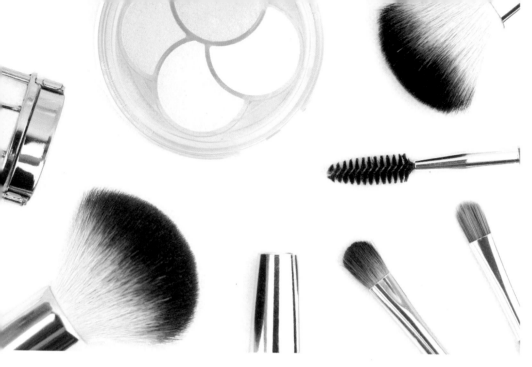

FACE POWDER

Arrowroot powder can also be used as a foundation. All you need to do is add nutmeg or cocoa powder until the shade matches your skin tone. Store in a reusable glass jar with a screw top lid (most arrowroot powders are sold in such receptacles).

EYELINER

Eyeliner has been used since around 10,000 BC, when the Egyptians and Mesopotamians wore it to help protect the delicate area around their eyes from the harsh desert sun. And of course, they wore it to enhance their natural eye beauty.

Ingredients
- ½ tsp activated charcoal
- Distilled water

Method
Mix together the charcoal and water to make a paste. Keep refrigerated and discard after three weeks. Use a narrow brush or cotton wool tip to apply. If the mixture is too watery, just add more charcoal. Use coconut oil to remove.

DEODORANT

The rise of natural deodorants over the past few years has been astonishing. This may be down to the negative coverage commercial deodorants have received – some media reports suggest that

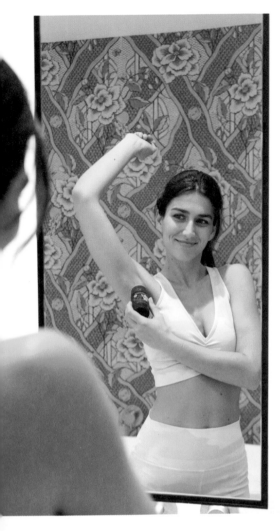

Natural deodorant is easy to make and a good alternative to commercial brands.
(Courtesy of The Creative Exchange/ Unsplash)

deodorants which contain aluminium can cause breast cancer. However, according to researchers, there is insufficient evidence to support the belief that using antiperspirants/deodorants increases the risk of getting breast cancer or Alzheimer's. The American Cancer Society (ACS) states that the main risk related to using these products is that they can cause skin irritation if a razor nick or cut becomes infected.

For some people though, regardless of what the researchers say, they prefer natural deodorants. There are many now available in health food stores (I particularly like the No Pong brand), although you can make your own.

A word of warning. If you are swapping from a commercial, or mass-produced deodorant it's advised you undergo an 'armpit detoxification'.

According to studies, people who switch from commercial deodorants to natural alternatives may experience rashes, excessive sweating and even an increased smell. It's thought that by using standard deodorants and antiperspirants you'll have built up an excess of bad bacteria in your armpit, which increases odour and causes more sweating.

To eliminate these issues, it's suggested you follow an 'armpit detox'. A word of advice – there is no evidence that following an armpit detox is any more effective than simply washing your underarms thoroughly morning and night with soap and water.

ARMPIT DETOX RECIPE

To help your body transition from man-made to natural deodorant you can try applying this mixture to your armpits. Use this mixture until there's no odour in your armpits or using natural deodorants do not irritate the skin.

Ingredients
1 tbsp bentonite clay
1 tbsp apple cider vinegar
1–2 tbsp water

Method

Mix the ingredients together until thick. Apply to your armpits and leave for around twenty minutes (you can begin slowly at three minutes and increase by a couple of minutes each day to build up to twenty minutes). Wash and remove the mixture with warm water.

NATURAL DEODORANT

This is a simple recipe which can be used as a natural deodorant. Best of all, you'll probably have these ingredients to hand.

Ingredients

3 tbsp coconut oil
2 tbsp baking soda
3 tbsp non-GMO corn starch

Method

Mix the ingredients thoroughly into a thick, stiff paste and spoon them into an empty bowl or jar. Allow to cool in the fridge until firm to the touch. Apply after showering or bathing.

SCENTED NATURAL DEODORANT

Another great recipe for your own deodorant is the one below. It combines a few more ingredients than the one above and has added fragrance, so I think it's worth the effort. Store in a reusable glass jar.

Ingredients

1/4 cup naturally-occurring bicarbonate of soda
1/4 cup bentonite clay or kaolin white clay
3½ tbsp coconut oil
4 drops lavender
4 drops rosemary

Method

In a medium-sized metal bowl mix together the bicarbonate of soda and clay, using wooden utensils. Mash in the coconut oil until well combined. Add the essential oils and store in jars or shallow tins. Allow to firm in a cool fridge and always store in a cool place. To use, rub a small amount onto dry armpits. Rub in, using your fingertips, until it becomes invisible. Apply again throughout the day if necessary.

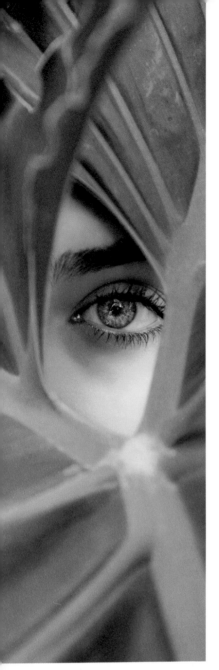

(Courtesy of Drew Graham)

FINAL WORD

I hope that you've become inspired to experiment with some of the recipes in this book and have enjoyed the pampering process!

Whether you decide to be 100 per cent natural or just follow some recipes for your weekly face and hair mask, the most important thing to remember is that beauty, and treatments, should be fun. So enjoy making your concoctions and experiment with some of your favourite recipes.

However many of the recipes you decide to adopt for daily, weekly, monthly or once-in-a-blue moon use, remember that it's important to be informed about the products you use on and in your skin. Do your research, read the labels, and always seek out an expert opinion for guidance and advice.

And don't forget the healing powers of food and what you eat and drink. A healthy, well-balanced diet, with regular exercise alongside natural beauty ingredients is truly the secret to a happy and beautiful life.

With thanks to Biome Australia for the ingredients to help make many of the recipes in this book.

Credit: DIY recipe and image courtesy of Australian eco store, Biome. Visit biome.com.au.

Acknowledgements

Thank you to my husband Conn Prosser for photographing my gorgeous niece Jessica for many of the pictures in this book. I couldn't have done this without you! And thank you to Jessica Bramley for allowing me to use her as a guinea pig and model – you truly are a natural beauty. And of course – thank you to my sons Zac and Joseph – beautiful souls inside and out.